GETTING STARTED IN GERIATRICS

A Guide for Medical Groups

By

Donna Onesian, MSW

and

Linda M. Bullock, MPH

Prepared by GeriMed of America, Inc.

With Support from the W.K. Kellogg Foundation of Battle Creek, Michigan.

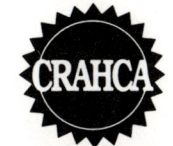

CENTER FOR RESEARCH
IN AMBULATORY
HEALTH CARE ADMINISTRATION

The research arm of the Medical Group Management Association
Denver, Colorado
1989

The preparation of this text was assisted by a grant from the W. K. Kellogg Foundation, Battle Creek, Michigan.

The opinions, conclusions, and proposals in the text are those of the authors and do not necessarily represent the views of the W. K. Kellogg Foundation, the Medical Group Management Association, or the Center for Research in Ambulatory Health Care Administration.

Copyright © 1989
Center for Research
in Ambulatory
Health Care Administration
1355 South Colorado Boulevard, Suite 900
Denver, Colorado 80222-3331
(303) 753-1111

ISBN 0-933948-98-0

No part of this book may be reproduced by any means or translated into a machine language without the written permission of the publisher.

Printed in the United States of America.

Table of Contents

About CRAHCA and MGMA vi
About GeriMed of America, Inc. vi
About the Authors vii
Acknowledgements viii
Introduction x
Preface — Facts on Aging Quiz xi

CHAPTER 1	**Geriatric Patient Relations**	1
	Patient Contact	1
	• Reception, Check-in and Scheduling	3
	• Volunteers	4
	• Telephone	5
	• Patient Satisfaction Questionnaire	6
	Transportation	8
	Billing	9
	• Medicare Assignment	9
	• Medicare Process	10
	• Medicare Parts A and B	10
	• Supplemental Insurance	11
CHAPTER 2	**Medical Considerations**	15
	Special Services	15
	• Options for the Hearing Impaired	15
	• Incontinence Clinic	16
	• Medication Monitoring	16
	Medical Equipment and Supplies	17
	• Supplies	18
	• Equipment	18
	• X-ray Equipment	18
	Medical Records	19
	• Demographics	20
	• Psycho/Social	20
	• Flow Sheet	20

i

CHAPTER 3	**Patient Education**		23
	Pamphlets		23
	Handouts		23
	Educational Classes		24
	Tips for Healthy Living Booklet		24
	Patient Handbook		24
	Healthy Lifestyle Approaches Booklet		25
	Newsletters		26
CHAPTER 4	**Referrals**		33
	Activities of Daily Living		33
		• Adult Day Care	34
		• Alzheimer's Assistance	34
		• Family Support Networks	34
		• Home Delivered Meals	34
		• Homemakers	34
		• Hospice	34
		• Respite Care - In Home	34
		• Respite Care - Outside Home	35
		• Senior Companions	35
		• Transportation	35
		• Meal Sites - Outside Home	36
	Housing		36
		• Independent Living	36
		• Assisted Living	36
		• Nursing Homes	36
		• Housecleaning/Homemaker Assistance	37
		• Utility Assistance	37
		• Weatherization	37
		• Yardwork Assistance	37
		• Grocery Delivery Services	37
	Social		37
		• Congregate Meal Programs	37
		• Employment Opportunities	38
		• Senior Centers/Community Centers	38
		• Telephone Reassurance Check	38
		• Volunteer Opportunities	39
	Mental Health		39
		• Mental Health Centers	39
		• Peer Counselor	39
		• Psychologist/Psychiatrist	39
		• Social Workers	39

CHAPTER 4
(continued)

- Support Groups 39
- Admission to a Psychiatric Hospital 40

Financial and Legal Assistance 40
- Food Stamps 41
- Insurance Counseling 41
- Legal Assistance 41
- Medicaid/Medi-Cal 41
- Medicare 41
- Social Security—Supplemental Security Income 41
- Social Security—Old Age Survivors and Disabled Insurance 41
- Social Services 41

Emergency or Abusive Assistance 41
- Adult Protective Services 42
- Crime Victim Assistance 42
- Emergency Care—Clothing, Financial, Food and Shelter 42
- 72-Hour Hold 42

Medical 42
- Services for the Blind 42
- Dental Care 42
- Nutritional and Diabetic Counseling 43
- Hearing Care 43
- Home Health Care 43
- Emergency Response Systems 43
- Substance Abuse Treatment 43
- Supportive Devices/Equipment/Supplies 43

CHAPTER 5

Geriatric Facility Design Considerations 44
Acoustics 44
Illumination/Glare 45
Use of Color/Pattern/Texture 46
Flooring 47
Carpeting 47
Grab Rails 48
Furniture 48
Entryway/Lobby 50
Art 50
Signage 51

CHAPTER 6

Marketing to the Geriatric Population 52
Demographics 52
- Identify the Potential Market 52
- Analyze the competition 52
- Strategies 52

CHAPTER 6 (continued)	Media	53
	• Print	53
	• Direct Mail	54
	• Articles	55
	• Radio	55
	• Television	56
	• Other Community Advertising	56
	The Little Extras	57
	• Health Fairs	57
	• Community Presentations	58
	• Cards	59
	• Special Patient Gifts	59
CHAPTER 7	**Geriatric Legal and Ethical Issues**	61
	Living Will	61
	Guardianship	62
	Revocation of Driver's License	64
CHAPTER 8	**Successful Geriatric Programs**	69
	Park Nicollet Medical Center	69
	• Friendly Caller Program	69
	• Over 50 and Fit Program	70
	• Nursing Home Program	70
	• Joint Venture with Local Hospital	70
	• Geriatric Assessment	71
	The Duluth Clinic, Limited	71
	• Health Education Presentations	71
	• The Gift of Memories Album	71
	• Healthy Lifestyle Approaches Workbook	71
	• Aging Awareness Questionnaire	72
	• Geriatric Assessment	72
	• Senior Expo Fair	72
	• Practicum Site	72
	The Honolulu Medical Group	72
	• Wellness Program	72
	• BestCare Supplemental Insurance Program	73
	• Geriatric Assessments	73
	• Honolulu Gerontology Program	73
	• Comprehensive Outpatient Rehabilitation Facility (CORF) Program	73
	• Educational Preceptorship and Practicum Placement Site	74
	• Geriatric Standards and Protocols	74

CHAPTER 8 (continued)		Carle Clinic Association	74
		• Geriatric Evaluation Clinic	74
		• Geriatric Consulting Service	74
		• Home Consultation Service	74
		• Wellness Program	74
		• Senior Companion Action Grant	75
		• Alzheimer's Grant	75
		• Focus Groups	75
		• Dementia Drug Trials	75
		• Carle Outreach Program for the Elderly (COPE)	75
Exhibits	1	HCFA Form #1561 - Health Insurance Benefit Agreement (Providers)	12
	2	HCFA Form #1561-A - Health Insurance Benefit Agreement (RHCs)	13
	3	HCFA Form #1500 - Health Insurance Claim	14
	4	Case Management Flow Sheet	22
	5	Sample Page - Tips for Healthy Living	27
	6	Patient Handbook Sample Pages	28
	7	Sample Page - Healthy Lifestyle Approaches	31
	8	Arbitron Rating Sheet	60
	9	Living Will	66
	10	Physicians Evaluation/Conservatorship	67
Appendices	1	Part B Medicare Insurance Carriers	76
	2	Referral Agencies	81
Bibliography			89
Index			92

About CRAHCA and MGMA

The Center for Research in Ambulatory Health Care Administration (CRAHCA) is a Section 501(c)(3) tax-exempt, charitable oranization as defined by the Internal Revenue Code. Founded in 1973, the purpose of CRAHCA is to improve ambulatory health care in general and group practice in particular through better administration by developing new and innovative publications; educational, research, and data services; and demonstration programs. The Center for Research is the research arm of the Medical Group Management Association (MGMA). The MGMA is a Section 501(c)(6) tax-exempt professional association. Founded in 1926, MGMA, which today is comprised of over 9,000 members in over 4,500 medical groups involving about 85,000 physicians, is the oldest and largest membership organization representing group practice administration. The MGMA serves its individual and organizational members, their patients, and promotes the group practice of medicine as an effective and efficient form of health care delivery.

About GeriMed of America, Inc.

GeriMed of America, Incorporated, is a private corporation based in Denver, Colorado, which develops, implements and manages comprehensive health care delivery systems enabling hospitals and medical groups to provide expanded services to senior citizens. As such, GeriMed consults with many providers and has cared for thousands of older adults in its ambulatory care facilities.

GeriMed's programs provide medical care and an array of senior programs at community based sites. Physicians, administrators, nurse practitioners, case managers, insurance counselors and ancillary personnel bring a team approach to senior care.

GeriMed's products and services include:
- The Senior Health Center—an outpatient Center providing comprehensive, patient-oriented service to the older adult
- Medicare Management Review—GeriMed's financial, operations and marketing specialists review existing programs and reimbursements to identify optimal reimbursement as well as service and marketing mix
- Program Development and Implementation—Assessment, Incontinence, Case Management
- Feasibility and Planning Analyses
- Older Adult Market Research
- Physical Plant Evaluation and Design
- Consulting

The world of health care has changed dramatically in recent years. GeriMed continues to grow and evolve with these changes, investing resources in staff and technologies to improve our client services.

About the Authors

Donna Onesian, MSW

Donna Onesian is the Case Management Coordinator for GeriMed of America. In this capacity, she is responsible for the development and operation of GeriMed's Case Management program.

Ms. Onesian has devised a complete assessment program which is in use at GeriMed's Senior Health Centers. She also assists with the daily case management duties at the Senior Health Center when needed. Ms. Onesian has contributed to several special consulting projects for GeriMed including development of a Patient Handbook and a booklet on tips for healthy living.

Ms. Onesian has a Bachelor degree in Gerontology from the University of Northern Colorado and a Master of Social Work degree from the University of Denver. Ms. Onesian is a volunteer for the Denver probate court and assists the court with guardianships for the elderly. She also serves on the Advisory Board for the Kinship Project of Colorado.

Linda Metzger Bullock, MPH

Linda Bullock, is the Administrative Director of the Mercy Senior Health Center in Denver. She was responsible for the planning and development of the Mercy Senior Health Center from the design and construction phase through full implementation. She also served as Project Manager for a special GeriMed consulting project designing a geriatric center of excellence in Calgary, Alberta, Canada.

Ms. Bullock has a Bachelor degree in Public Policy from Pomona College and a Master degree in Public Health from Columbia University. Before joining GeriMed, she held various marketing and consulting positions as well as a Congressional Internship to the late Congressman Claude Pepper, former Chairman of the House Select Committee on Aging. Ms. Bullock currently serves as President of Older Adult Service and Information System (OASIS) in Denver.

Acknowledgements

The Center for Research in Ambulatory Care Administration, the research arm of the Medical Group Management Association, would like to express its gratitude to the W. K. Kellogg Foundation, Battle Creek, Michigan, for its support in funding the development of "A Demonstration Project Integrating Gerontology Program Models in Medical Group Settings." This project consists of three major components:

1. The publication of manuals dealing with case management, patient assessment, a medical group service assessment, and this book.
2. The production of two videotapes: "In Our Age—The Older Patient," and "New Age Volunteers: Seniors Helping Seniors."
3. Education programs which outline some of the services physician practices may wish to institute in meeting the needs of its elderly patients.

Appreciation is extended to the Project Task Force which aided in establishing a direction for the development of each of the above components. Members of the Task Force include:

Oscar Kurren, PhD
Co-Principal Investigator for the Project
Honolulu Medical Group, Inc.
Honolulu, Hawaii

Harvey Anderson
The Duluth Clinic, Limited
Duluth, Minnesota

Candace Bruno
The Duluth Clinic, Limited
Duluth, Minnesota

Karen Buck, FACMGA
Southwestern Eye Center
Mesa, Arizona

Cheryl Crowley, PhD
Carle Clinic Association
Urbana, Illinois

Neill Fishman
Park Nocollet Medical Center
Minneapolis, Minnesota

Arlynna Howell-Livingston
Honolulu Medical Group, Inc.
Honolulu, Hawaii

Sharon Marx, MD
Park Nicollet Medical Center
Minneapolis, Minnesota

Sandra Wood Reifsteck, FACMGA
Carle Clinic Association
Urbana, Illinois

The Center for Research would also like to acknowledge the efforts of members of the staff who were involved in the implementation of the funded project.

Mary Alice Krill, PhD
Administrative Director
and Director of Research

Anna M. Bergstrom
Project Director

Mary Jo Ross
Administrative Assistant

Patricia J. Doty
Word Processing Clerk

For further information about the project, please contact the Center for Research at the address shown on the inside of the title page.

GeriMed Staff

Carolyn Hoy, Contributing Author and Editor
Debra Reinberg, Editor
Edward B. Daniels, Editor
Suzanne Houck, Consultant
Lori Mitchell, Consultant

Mercy Senior Health Center Staff

Professional Consultants

Erica Wood, Associate Director of the American Bar Association Commission on Legal Problems of the Elderly

Kathie Regan, Unit Director Mobility Services, Office of Vocational Rehabilitation

Shirley Neitlich, Public Information Specialist, Society for the Right to Die

Pamela Venturi, Vice President - Reich Communications

Peter Wisdom, Social Worker, Beth Israel Gero Psych Unit

Introduction

The number of physician visits by the elderly is expected to increase by 47 percent between 1980 and the year 2000. Many of these older patients have special needs; most have at least one chronic condition, and many have multiple conditions such as arthritis (50 percent), hypertension (39 percent), hearing impairments (30 percent) and heart conditions (26 percent). Persons aged 65 and over average eight physician visits per year, compared with five visits per year for persons under 65.

The dilemma for individual physicians and medical groups is that this increase in the number of older patients, many with special needs, has been accompanied by decreasing reimbursement and increasing regulatory requirements. For most, reducing the number of older patients is not an option. Instead, medical groups must find ways to profitably meet the needs of an older population and turn this problem into an opportunity. Medical groups who can successfully provide care to older patients will find tremendous growth potential and an appreciative base of patients and of families.

This guide was designed to assist medical groups in their efforts to provide quality care to the growing number of seniors. Older adults have special needs, and by meeting those needs medical groups will enhance their ability to attract and maintain a large base of older patients. They will also provide an environment where medical care can be rendered more efficiently and more profitably. The understanding, compliant patient with an effective social support structure is easier to manage and less demanding of physician time than a confused, recalcitrant patient with nowhere else to turn for support and understanding.

This guide provides a broad range of ideas and recommendations in areas which include patient relations, special services, medical equipment, medical records, patient education, referrals, facility design, marketing, legal and ethical issues and several case histories. It also contains numerous references to agencies which can be contacted for further, more in-depth information on the many topics discussed.

It is important to note that no one medical group will be able to implement all of the ideas and recommendations contained in this guide. Smaller practices, for example, will be limited in their ability to hire and train additional personnel. But even they should be able to gain a better understanding of the needs of their older patients, and to pick up a few ideas and concepts which will be of benefit to patient and provider alike.

Preface
Facts On Aging, A Short Quiz

The following quiz about aging was adapted from Dr. Erdman Palmore's book *The Facts on Aging Quiz*. Whenever possible, statistics were updated from his original documentation to reflect current information.

The quiz was developed to clarify and identify misconceptions about aging and it can be used to stimulate group discussion. Clinics can administer the quiz to their employees and volunteers, as The Duluth Clinic, Limited, in Minnesota does, to help dispel many of the myths associated with aging and to encourage discussion.

T F 1. The majority of older people (past age 65) are senile (i.e., defective memory, disoriented or demented).

T F 2. All five senses tend to weaken in old age.

T F 3. Most older people have no interest in, nor capacity for, sexual relations.

T F 4. Physical strength tends to decline in old age.

T F 5. The majority of older people feel miserable most of the time.

T F 6. Most older people cannot work as effectively as younger workers.

T F 7. Aged drivers have fewer accidents per person than drivers under age 65.

T F 8. The majority of old people are unable to adapt to change.

T F 9. Over three-fourths of the aged are healthy enough to carry out their normal activities.

T F 10. The majority of older people are socially isolated.

T F 11. Older people have more injuries in the home than persons under 65.

T F 12. Older people tend to react slower than younger people.

T F 13. Medicare pays over half of the medical expenses for the aged.

Used by permission of the publisher, Springer Publishing Company, Inc., New York, NY 10012, from "The FActs on AGing Quiz," Parts 1 and 2, pp. 3-19, in *The FActs on Aging Quiz* by Erdman B. Palmore, PhD. Copyright 1988.

T F 14. The majority of older people are seldom irritated or angry.

T F 15. The aged have higher rates of criminal victimization than persons under 65.

T F 16. There are equal numbers of widows and widowers among the aged.

T F 17. More older persons (over 65) have chronic illnesses that limit their activity than younger persons.

T F 18. The majority of aged live alone.

T F 19. Supplemental Security Income guarantees a minimum income for needy adults.

T F 20. Older persons who reduce their activity tend to be happier than those who remain active.

Answers

1. *False.* The majority of people aged 65 or over are not senile; that is, they do not have defective memory, nor are they disoriented or demented. Only about 2 percent of persons aged 65 or over are institutionalized with a primary diagnosis of psychiatric illness. All community studies of psychopathology among the aged agree that less than 10 percent have significant or severe mental illness and another 10 percent to 32 percent have mild to moderate mental impairment; but the majority are without impairment.

2. *True.* All five senses do tend to decline in old age. Most studies of taste and smell show that taste and odor sensitivity decrease with age, although some of these decreases may be the result of other factors, such as disease, drugs and smoking. Nearly all studies of touch, hearing and vision agree that these senses tend to decline in old age.

3. *False.* The majority of persons past age 65 continue to have both interest in and capacity for sexual relations. Masters and Johnson (1966) found that the capacity for satisfying sexual relations usually continues into the seventies and eighties for healthy couples. A recent survey of the elderly found that most indicated sex after 60 was as satisfying or more satisfying than when younger.

4. *True.* Physical strength does tend to decline in old age. Physiological, biochemical, anatomic and histocytological measurements of muscle all exhibit decreased levels with age from about the third decade. About one-third of the muscle mass is lost by age 80.

5. *False.* The majority of older people do not feel miserable most of the time. Studies of happiness, morale and life satisfaction either find no significant difference by age groups or find about

one-fifth to one-third of the aged score "low" on various happiness or morale scales. A national survey found that less than a fourth of persons 65 or over reported that "This is the dreariest time of my life;" while a majority said, "I am just as happy as when I was younger."

6. *False.* Despite declines in perception and reaction speed under laboratory conditions among the general aged population, studies of older workers (those able to continue employment) under actual working conditions generally show that they perform as well as young workers, if not better than younger workers, on most measures. Consistency of output tends to increase by age. In addition, older workers have less job turnover, less accidents and less absenteeism than younger workers. About 3.1 million older Americans were in the labor force (working or actively seeking work) in 1987.

7. *True.* Drivers over age 65 do have fewer accidents per person than drivers under age 65. Older drivers have about the same accident rate per person as middle-aged drivers, but a much lower rate than drivers under age 30.

8. *False.* Older people are more adaptable to change due to a lifetime of experience with change. Today's 70 year old has lived through a depression, a world war, the birth of the nuclear age, and a host of other technological breakthroughs. Stubbornness is a character trait brought into old age, not created by it.

9. *True.* About 80 percent of the aged are healthy enough to engage in their normal activities. About 5 percent of those over age 65 are institutionalized and another 15 percent say they are unable to engage in their major activity (such as work or housework) because of chronic conditions. This leaves 80 percent who are able to engage in their major activity.

10. *False.* The majority of old people are not socially isolated. About two-thirds live with their spouse or family. Only about 4 percent of the elderly are extremely isolated, and most of these have had lifelong histories of withdrawal. Most elders have close relatives within easy visiting distance and contact between them is relatively frequent.

11. *False.* Older persons have less injuries in the home than younger persons: twelve injuries per 100 persons over 65 per year compared to 14 injuries for persons under 65. The injury rate is especially high for children under 6: 26 per 100.

12. *True.* The reaction time of most older people tends to be slower than that of younger people. This is one of the best documented facts about the aged on record. It appears to be true regardless of the kind of reaction that is measured.

13. *False.* Medicare pays less than half of the medical expenses for the aged. In 1984, Medicare payments covered 48.8 percent of the personal health expenditures of the aged. Medicaid covered an additional 13 percent (among the "medically indigent"), other public programs

(such as the Veteran's Administration) covered another 6 percent, and the remaining was paid by private insurance or "out of pocket."

14. *True.* The majority of old people do say they are seldom irritated or angry. The Duke Second Longitudinal Study found that 90 percent of persons aged 65 or over said they were never angry during the past week. About three-fourths of the aged in a Kansas City Study said they were never or hardly ever angry.

15. *False.* The aged actually have lower rates of criminal victimization than those under 65. Persons over 65 have substantially lower victimization rates in nearly all categories of personal crime: rape, robbery, assault and personal theft. The only category for which the rate for older persons is even equal that of younger persons is "personal larceny with contact" (which includes purse-snatching and pick-pocketing) and this category accounts for less than three percent of all personal crimes. When all personal crimes are added together, persons over 65 have a victimization rate that is less than one-fourth that of all persons over age 12 (31 per 1,000 compared to 128 per 1,000).

16. *False.* There are over five times as many widows as widowers among the aged. This is the result of several factors: women tend to marry men older than themselves; women tend to live longer than men; and widows do not remarry as often as do widowers, partly because of the scarcity of eligible widowers.

17. *True.* More persons over 65 have chronic illnesses that limit their activity (46 percent) than younger persons (12 percent). The discrepancy is similar for the percentages with chronic illnesses that limit their major activity: 39 percent for those 65 and older, and 10 percent for those under 65.

18. *False.* The majority of aged do not live alone. In 1987, for example, 16 percent of men 65 or over lived alone and 41.6 percent of women 65 or over lived alone. The majority lived with their spouse (75 percent of men, 39 percent of women). Another 7 percent of men and 18 percent of women live with relatives other than a spouse.

19. *True.* About 3.5 million elderly persons, representing 12.2 percent of the elderly population, were below the poverty level in 1987. Supplemental Security Income (SSI) is a program that provides a modest monthly cash benefit to eligible low income persons. The monthly Federal SSI payment in 1989 can be up to $388 a month for an individual and $573 a month for a couple depending on other income sources.

20. *False.* Older persons who disengage from active roles do not tend to be happier than those who remain active. On the contrary, most surveys and longitudinal studies have found that those who remain active tend to be happier than those who disengage, although some studies found no relationship between activity and happiness.

CHAPTER 1
Geriatric Patient Relations

Patient relations begins with the person-to-person care administered by medical office personnel. They set the tone for the visit and potential subsequent appointments. With seniors especially, the warmth that pervades the reception area is one of the major ingredients of a successful practice.

Just as the family physician of yesterday knew his patients and their families, front desk personnel should learn about their patients and families. Calling the son of a heart patient when his mother neither shows up for an appointment nor answers the telephone, surprising Viola with a birthday cake on her 105th birthday, and giving Mrs. Lopez a hug and extending condolences on the death of her husband are little things which can make a big difference.

Patient Contact

The staff must remember that when they interact with an older person, they are communicating with someone who might have a combination of physical disabilities, such as failing eyesight, hearing loss, limited mobility and slower reaction time. By remembering to be patient, considerate and caring, the staff can create a positive experience for these patients and for themselves.

Older people require special considerations when providing medical care. As people age, they visit their physician more often for conditions which may be chronic and non-curable. Often the visit is for comfort and understanding more than for medical expertise. Older patients experience more changes than at any other time in their lives. These changes include losses, such as loss of health and physical ability, loss of friends and loved ones, loss of income and loss of independence. These losses contribute to increased stress levels.

The staff of the medical office (including the physician) can provide support and encouragement and increase a patient's responsiveness by following these techniques:

- The rhythm while interacting with the elderly is half-time. It is important to understand that more time should be allocated for this age group.

- Sit or squat when talking with seated patients. It is important for the older patient to see the speaker on an eye-to-eye level.

- Sit by the patient rather than behind a desk. Remember, the patient will often look for facial cues from the speaker.

- Lean toward the patient and listen to what they have to say.

- Use eye contact when the patient speaks so he or she knows staff is listening.

- It is important for the patient to know the staff person cares. A gentle touch at appropriate times demonstrates support and understanding.

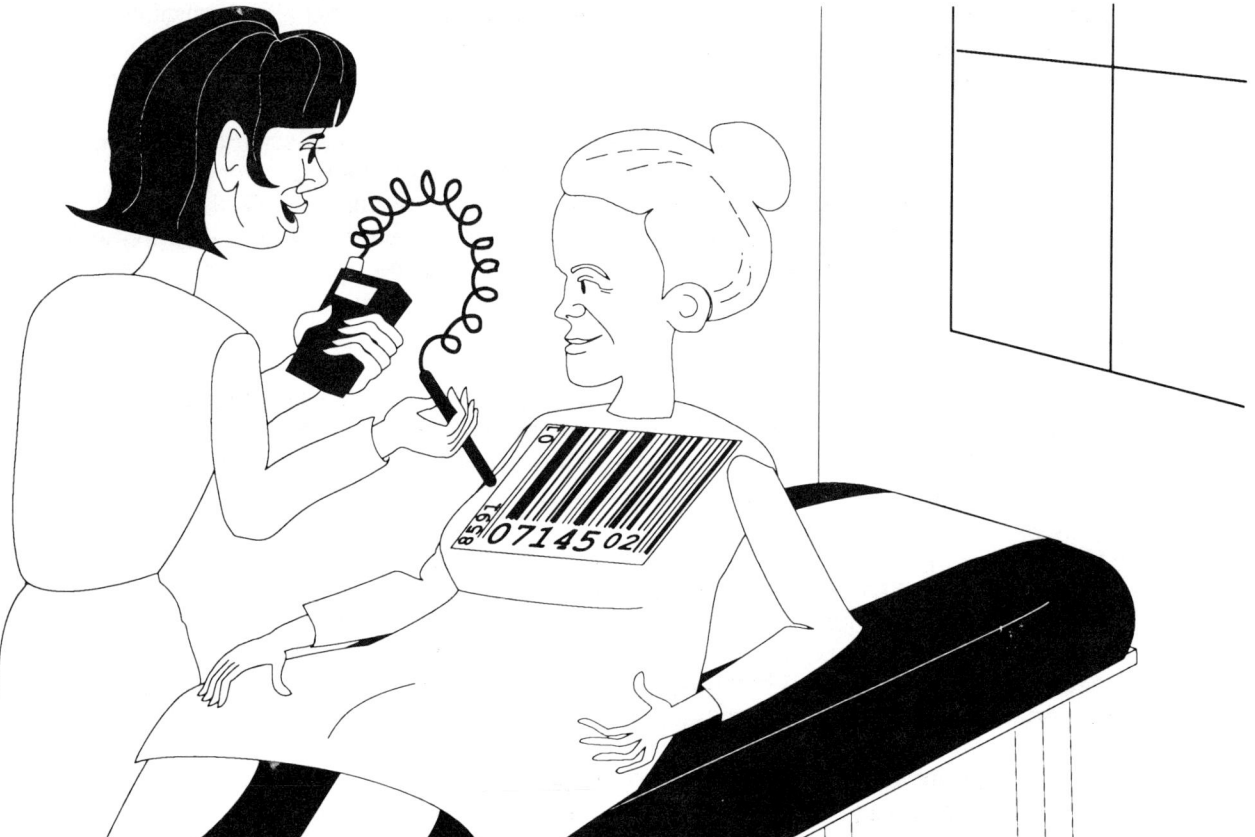

"This is another technique the clinic has devised to make your stay here less impersonal and degrading."

- Be clear when discussing medical concerns with the patient. Try not to use too much medical terminology.

- When the staff person is not sure the patient has understood, ask the patient to repeat what was explained, especially concerning instructions with procedures and medications. In most cases, it is best to write down instructions or staff may suggest that the patient take notes to refer to later.

- Become familiar with non-medical as well as medical aspects of the patient's life, such as living situations and family support. It is appropriate for physicians and other staff members to refer patients to community agencies for their non-medical needs. Often, by not addressing these other issues, the medical issues can get worse. (See CHAPTER 4 for information about referrals on non-medical issues.)

- Offer positive reinforcement when possible. For example, congratulate the patient on his or her 5-pound weight loss. Show understanding of the difficulty of the process and encourage him or her to lose additional poundage by the next visit.

Reception, Check-in and Scheduling. The medical office staff is responsible for greeting the patients, managing the patient flow during the office's operating hours and scheduling. It is important that every employee interacting with older patients use the following simple considerations:

- Each patient should be greeted upon arrival. A smile and a nod will suffice if the reception desk is extremely busy.

- Some patients need assistance opening the front door. Gladly aid those patients who need help.

- Older patients should be greeted respectfully by their last name, unless they have asked to be addressed otherwise.

- Use eye contact and give the patient your full attention.

- If possible, place a chair at the check-in desk and at the scheduling desk so the patient can sit down while filling out forms. It may be difficult for a more frail patient to stand, even for only a minute.

- If the office has a high desk or if the patient is wheelchair-bound, walk around the desk to the patient. Do not stand over the patient. Either sit next to the patient or squat down to their eye level.

- Address the patient directly — do not talk about the patient to the person who may be assisting him or her.

- After giving a patient forms to complete, remain within hearing distance in case they have any questions.

- To aid a hearing impaired patient, look squarely at the patient while talking to him or her. It is important that the patient be able to see your facial expressions.

- Staff may need to assist some patients to and from the bathroom.

- Order magazines and large print books for the reception area. Provide a magnifying glass for those patients with weak eyesight.

- Instructional forms, including appointment cards, which are filled out or handed out to the patient should be printed in extra large print (at least 14 point) for easier reading.

Volunteers. Volunteers can be beneficial to any physician practice. They expand staff resources without increasing costs. Older people and student interns are usually the most interested in volunteering to assist within a physician office. To seek out volunteers:

- Recruit patients from the practice itself.

- Post notices at local senior centers.

- Make appeals during presentations to senior groups or associations.

- Place advertisements in senior newspapers.

- Contact local colleges and high schools.

- Word of mouth — let staff and patients know the practice needs volunteers.

Volunteers can perform a variety of duties depending on their areas of interest and background. Volunteers can be utilized to:

- Assist secretary and receptionist with phones, transportation arrangements, and registration.

- Assist billing department wherever needed.

- Aid in the comfort and well being of waiting patients.

- Prepare mailings.

- If background permits, assist medical staff with various duties.

- Help patients locate community resources.

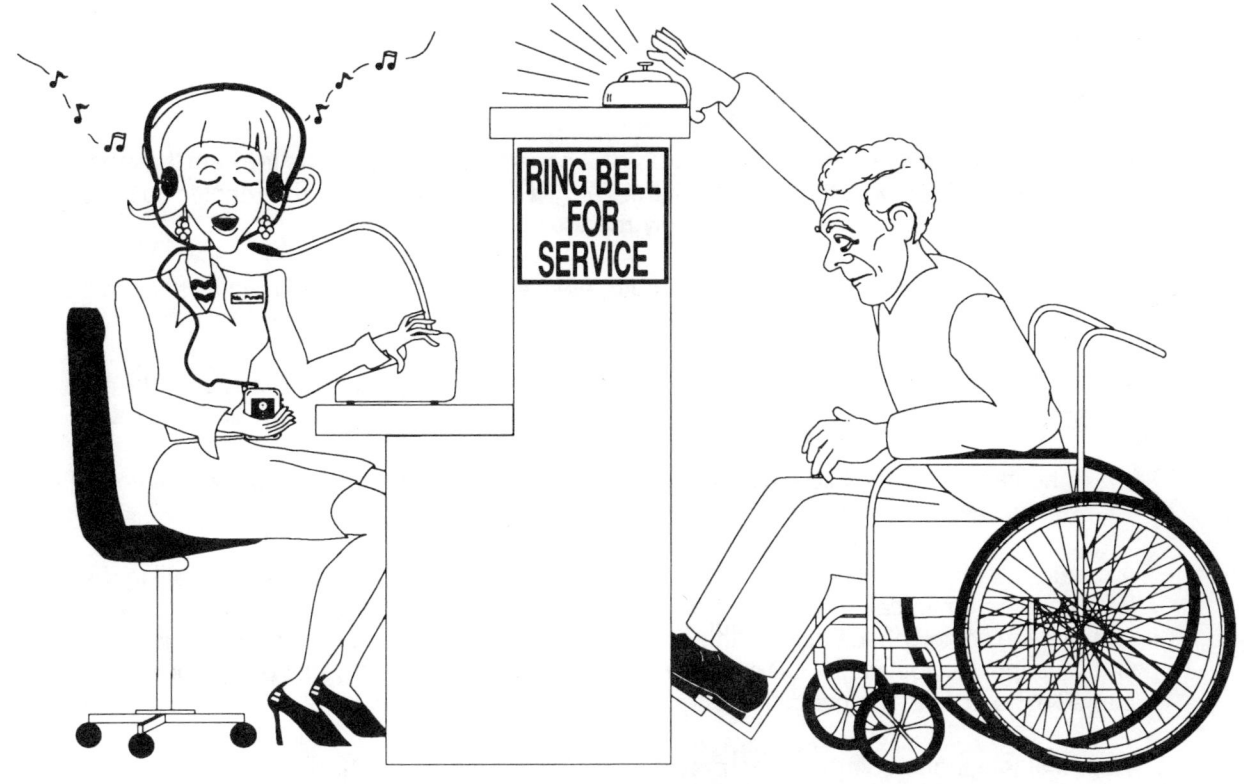

"I think the phones are on the fritz. I keep hearing these funny bells."

Telephone. The person calling the medical office cannot see the facial expression of the person with whom he or she is talking. The sound of the receptionist's voice must convey the impression of warmth and caring. The receptionist should always use the following phone courtesies:

- Identify yourself: "Good morning/afternoon, Dr. _____'s office. This is _____."

- Be patient with the older callers as it may take them more time to explain their needs.

- Speak clearly and simply; lower the tone of your voice and speak a little louder for those who are hard of hearing.

- Listen carefully.

- Keep a smile in your voice.

- Older people may be lonely and may use the opportunity on the phone to share their thoughts. If time permits, talk with the patient. However, in a busy practice, it is important to be diplomatic in ending the conversation in a timely manner.

- If the caller must wait, say "Will you hold, please?" Be sure to wait for an answer, in case it is an emergency.

- If the caller must wait long, keep in touch by returning to the line and advising the caller of progress and continued attention.

- If the call is to schedule an appointment, repeat the time and date of the appointment and wait for the caller to write it down.

A physician's office which sees many hearing impaired patients should consider installing a special telephone communication system. Teletypewriters (TTY's) or TDD's (Telecommunication Device for the Deaf) are telephone devices that enable the hearing impaired to communicate via telephone lines. A paper printout or an LCD screen must be installed at each end. One party types a message into a keyboard and the message is transmitted to the other party.

The local telephone company can provide information regarding the services available in your state. Many phone companies have a Center for Disabled Customers or the local Deaf Association may be of assistance. Some states charge a surcharge to all customers that is placed in a general fund to purchase TTY/TDD devices for the hearing impaired. Other states may require individuals to qualify as low-income in order to receive devices free of charge. If purchased, TTY/TDD devices are $200 to $700 per unit. Some states provide a relay service with an intermediary that receives the messages from the hearing impaired and then transmits them through normal telephone procedures. Most local companies provide discounts for TTY/TDD long-distance services because of the extended length of time required to communicate.

Patient Satisfaction Questionnaire. A patient satisfaction questionnaire can be used to obtain a patient's feelings, perceptions, attitudes and judgments about the practice. It can also be used to evaluate the staff and the services provided. A survey can be distributed in person, it can be mailed, or a phone survey can be conducted. The physicians and staff should discuss what questions would be relevant to the practice.

Below are some questions which may be included:

1. How would you rate the length of time you had to wait

    a) to get an appointment

    EXCELLENT   GOOD   FAIR   POOR

    b) in the waiting room

    EXCELLENT   GOOD   FAIR   POOR

    c) in the exam room

    EXCELLENT   GOOD   FAIR   POOR

2. Was the staff at the clinic courteous and professional during your visit?

    YES   NO   COMMENTS: _____

3. Have you experienced difficulty with the billing process? If yes, would you like assistance with your billing and insurance questions?

4. Do transportation problems ever keep you from visiting the clinic?

5. Are there any subjects or topics which you would like to see included in our clinic newsletter?

6. What can we do to better serve you at our office?

Questionnaires can be given out at each visit or over a selected period of time. Once they are tallied, problems and successes can be identified and shared with the entire staff.

CRAHCA/Kellogg Gerontology Project Patient Questionnaire.

Hello, my name is _____, and I'm calling from the _____. We're asking some of our patients to tell us about the care and services they received at _____ and I'd like to ask you some questions about this. Would you mind taking 5 minutes to help us.?

	Strongly Disagree	Disagree	Agree	Strongly Agree
1. Overall, I was satisfied with the care I received in the _____.	1	2	3	4
2. The services provided by __ helped me with my need/problem.	1	2	3	4
3. The staff were very responsive to my needs.	1	2	3	4
4. Participation in the _____ was worth the fee that was charged.	1	2	3	4
5. I would recommend the _____ to others.	1	2	3	4

6. Do you have any comments you would like to make about the _____?
7. Are there other services you would like to see developed at _____?

Transportation

Many older people no longer drive, but instead depend upon friends and relatives for transportation. Scheduling physician appointments around a friend or relative's schedule can often be difficult to coordinate. Therefore, the staff at the front desk should have suggestions for alternate means of transportation for their older patients. There are many local and private transportation services:

- Many cities offer rides for elderly and disabled people either for a donation or on a fee-for-service basis. Look under "Senior Services" or "Transportation" in the Yellow Pages for "Senior Rides." Keep phone numbers and brochures handy at the front desk and in the waiting room.

- Talk to local taxi companies about their policies on senior discounts.

- Provide local bus schedules at the front desk and know enough about the neighborhood to be able to suggest possible routes.

- Area county social service offices often provide transportation to and from medical appointments for patients on Medicaid or Medi-Cal.

Some practices may be large enough to justify the purchase of a van or to share a van with another office. A patient survey can be performed to determine how many people would use a van service. The purchase of a van is an expensive investment. The practice may not recoup its investment over the life of the van unless new patients are attracted because of the transportation service offered. Costs associated with a van include:
— Driver's salary
— Insurance
— Yearly registration and purchase of license plates
— Fuel
— Maintenance and tune-ups
— Wheelchair ramp (an electric lift is more costly to install and maintain)
— Lettering needed to print the name of the clinic on the van for advertising

Additional points to consider if the practice purchases a van:

- Provide a step stool to assist patients into and out of the van.

- Keep a transportation schedule in a notebook at the front desk. The person responsible for scheduling appointments should also schedule transportation needs to ensure the most efficient use of the van.

- Provide a daily schedule to the driver with room to record mileage for tax purposes.

- If van transportation is offered as a free service, place a donation box in the reception area. Some people may want to contribute to their rides.

Billing

Many older patients are overwhelmed and confused by Medicare and supplemental insurance paperwork. If possible, one person from the office staff should be designated and trained to explain the billing process and the complexities of Medicare insurance programs. (Contact the State Department of Insurance for information on local advocacy programs.) A written explanation and diagram of the billing system should be available to help the patient understand the process. And, finally, a quiet area should be designated where billing issues can be discussed in private.

Often inquiries are received regarding Medicare's assignment method of billing. The following is an explanation of Medicare assignment and the process.

Medicare Assignment. Medicare Assignment was designed to be an easier method of billing for both the physician and the patient. It is simpler for physicians because they can bill one carrier (the Medicare contractor) and be assured that the Medicare payment will come directly to them. (See Appendix 1, List of Carriers by State). It is easier for patients because they do not have to worry about submitting paperwork to Medicare. By accepting assignment, physicians agree to accept the Medicare-approved amount. Medicare will then pay the provider (the physician) 80 percent of the approved amount. The remaining 20 percent may be billed to either the patient or the supplemental insurance carrier.

The following diagram may clarify the process further:

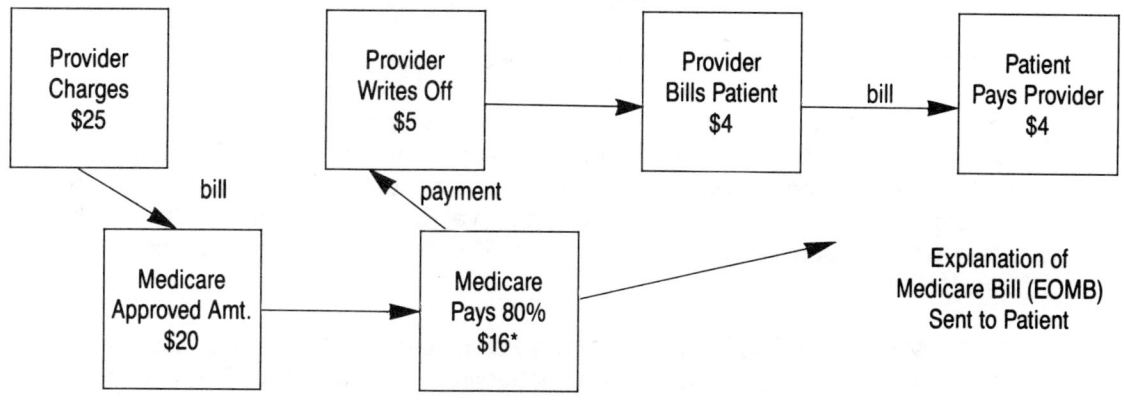

* if deductible has been met

Medicare requires physicians to participate, or to "accept assignment" on all of their Medicare patients in order to receive all the benefits that Medicare assignment provides. Physicians do have the option to accept assignment on an individual basis; however, they may not be eligible to receive all benefits. These benefits (both to the physician and to the patient) include:

- The staff bills Medicare directly, eliminating the need for patients to handle the bills.

- Medicare pays the providers' office directly. Patients seen by physicians who do not accept assignment are responsible for billing Medicare. It may be difficult to collect the payment from the patient in a timely and efficient manner. Therefore, some physicians who do not accept assignment request payment at the time of service.

- Claims can be electronically transmitted directly to the Medicare contractor.

- As incentives to participate, participating physicians' names are published in directories and their names are also available through toll-free telephone lines.

Medicare Process. For physicians interested in accepting assignment, a participation agreement HCFA form 1561 or HCFA form 1561-A for rural health clinics may be submitted to the Secretary of Health and Human Services through the applicable state carrier. (See Exhibit 1 on page 12 and Exhibit 2 on page 13.) Points covered in the agreement include:
— stated willingness to be a participating physician
— acceptance of the Medicare allowed amount as payment in full
— agreement to accept 80 percent of the Medicare determined approved amount as payment from the patient's primary insurance for all Medicare patients
— agreement to process claims through Medicare for all Medicare patients, using HCFA form 1500 (See Exhibit 3 on page 14.)

Medicare Parts A and B. Medicare is divided into two parts:

Part A - HOSPITAL INSURANCE. Medicare Part A covers inpatient care including Skilled Nursing Facility benefits. Under Part A, Medicare pays for all acute care hospital costs, excluding a $560 deductible each year. In Skilled Nursing Facilities, the patient is responsible for $25.50/day for the first eight days. Medicare will then pay for all covered services from the 9th through the 150th day provided the patient is receiving skilled care. Medicare Part A also provides for home health and hospice care.

Part B - MEDICAL INSURANCE. Medicare Part B covers physicians' services, outpatient hospital care, x-rays, lab charges and many other services and supplies. After an annual deductible of $75.00, Medicare will pay 80 percent of the remaining approved charges for any covered service.

Supplemental Insurance. Supplemental or "Medigap" insurance is private health care insurance that helps pay for medical expenses not covered by Medicare. Supplemental policies benefit patients by reducing out-of-pocket expenses for health care. Supplemental insurance is offered by private insurance companies which insure approximately 42 percent of the over-65 population.

For supplemental insurance to work, the patient must also have Medicare Parts A and B. Usually if Medicare approves a covered service, so will the supplement. However, if Medicare denies a service, so will the supplement. Supplementals vary widely in the coverage of charges for physician's services and outpatient care (provided by Part B). They offer benefits that cover from 20 percent to 100 percent of the charges that Medicare does not cover. In addition, some supplementals offer more coverage than others, specifically for services such as eye care and prescription drug coverage.

It is important for office personnel to be familiar with supplemental policies and to understand how various supplemental policies differ. Personnel should:

- Discuss supplemental policies with patients who do not carry a supplemental policy.

- If the physician accepts assignment, bill the supplemental directly after Medicare has paid to insure payments rather than relying on the patient to submit paperwork.

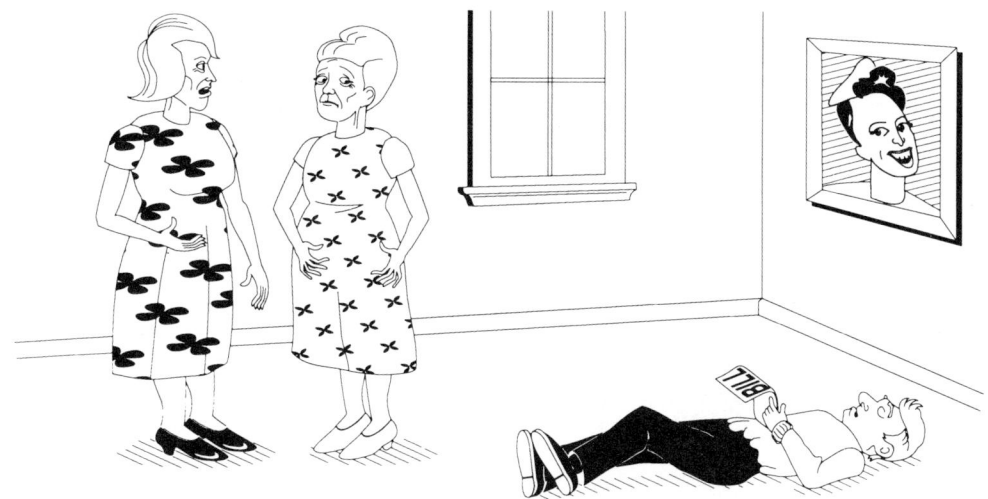

"It wasn't the size of the bill that made him faint - it was that it was actually covered by Medicare."

Exhibit 1

HCFA-1561—HEALTH INSURANCE BENEFIT AGREEMENT (PROVIDERS)

> Form HCFA-1561 is reproduced from the *State Operations Manual*,

HEALTH INSURANCE BENEFIT AGREEMENT
(Agreement Pursuant to Section 1866 of the
Social Security Act and 42 CFR 400 et seq.)

In order to receive payment under Title XVIII of the Social Security Act, _____ D/B/A _____ as the provider of services, agrees:

(a) not to charge except as permitted by section 1866(a)(2) of the Act and pertinent regulations, any person for items or services precluded by section 1866(a)(1).

(b) to return any moneys incorrectly collected from any person or to dispose of overpayments as specified in regulations;

(c) to notify promptly the Health Care Financing Administration of the employment of any individual in a managerial, accounting, auditing or similar capacity who was employed by the Fiscal Intermediary within the previous 12 months.

This agreement, upon submission by the provider of services of acceptable assurance of compliance with Title VI of the Civil Rights Act of 1964, section 504 of the Rehabilitation Act of 1973 as amended, and upon acceptance by the Secretary of Health and Human Services, shall be binding on the provider of services and the Secretary. The agreement may be terminated by either party in accordance with the provisions of section 1866(b)(1) and (2) of the Act and pertinent regulations. In the event of termination, the obligations of the Secretary to make payments to the provider of services shall be abrogated as stated in 1866(b)(3), (4), and (5) of the Act and pertinent regulations.

This agreement will be effective as determined by the Health Care Financing Administration, the Secretary's delegate.

In the event of a transfer of ownership, this agreement is assigned to the new owner, subject to the conditions specified in this agreement and pertinent regulations.

FOR PROVIDER OF SERVICES BY:	Accepted by the Secretary of Health and Human Services by:
NAME	NAME
TITLE	TITLE
DATE	DATE

Form HCFA-1561 (4-80)

Exhibit 2

HCFA-1561A—HEALTH INSURANCE BENEFITS AGREEMENT (RHCs)

> Form HCFA-1561A is reproduced from the *State Operations Manual,*

HEALTH INSURANCE BENEFITS AGREEMENT
(Agreement with Rural Health Clinic Pursuant to Section 1861 of the Social Security Act)

For the purpose of establishing eligibility for payment under Title XVIII of the Social Security Act, _____ hereinafter referred to as the rural health clinic, hereby agrees

(A) to maintain compliance with the conditions set forth in Part 481 of Chapter IV, Title 42 of the Code of Federal Regulations, and to report promptly to the Health Care Financing Administration any failure to do so.

(B) not charge a Medicare beneficiary or any other person for items and services for which the beneficiary would be entitled to have payment made in accordance with Part 405 of Chapter IV, Title 42 of the Code of Federal Regulations, except for any deductible and coinsurance amounts for which the beneficiary is liable as set forth herein.

(C) to refund as promptly as possible any moneys incorrectly collected from a beneficiary or from someone on his or her behalf.

(D) to accept beneficiaries for care and treatment without limitations, except as it may impose on all other persons.

(E) to have acceptable assurance of compliance with the requirements of Title VI of the Civil Rights Act of 1964.

This agreement, upon submission by the rural health clinic and upon acceptance for filing by the Secretary of Health, Education, and Welfare, shall be binding on the rural health clinic and the Secretary. The agreement may be terminated by either party in accordance with regulations. In the event of termination, payment will not be available for rural health clinic services furnished on or after the effective date of termination.

This agreement shall become effective on the date specified below by the Secretary or the Secretary's delegate.

For Supplier of Services by:	Accepted for Secretary of Health, Education, and Welfare by:
NAME	NAME
TITLE	TITLE
DATE	DATE

Form HCFA-1561A (9-79)

Exhibit 3

HEALTH INSURANCE CLAIM FORM

(CHECK APPLICABLE PROGRAM BLOCK BELOW)

☐ MEDICARE (MEDICARE NO.) ☐ MEDICAID (MEDICAID NO.) ☐ CHAMPUS (SPONSOR'S SSN) ☐ CHAMPVA (VA FILE NO.) ☐ FECA BLACK LUNG (SSN) ☐ OTHER (CERTIFICATE SSN)

PATIENT AND INSURED (SUBSCRIBER) INFORMATION

1 PATIENT'S NAME (LAST NAME, FIRST NAME, MIDDLE INITIAL)

2 PATIENT'S DATE OF BIRTH

3 INSURED'S NAME (LAST NAME, FIRST NAME, MIDDLE INITIAL)

4 PATIENT'S ADDRESS (STREET, CITY, STATE, ZIP CODE)

5 PATIENT'S SEX — MALE ☐ ☐ FEMALE

6 INSURED'S I.D. NO. (FOR PROGRAM CHECKED ABOVE, INCLUDE ALL LETTERS)

7 PATIENT'S RELATIONSHIP TO INSURED — SELF ☐ SPOUSE ☐ CHILD ☐ OTHER ☐

8 INSURED'S GROUP NO. (OR GROUP NAME OR FECA CLAIM NO.)

☐ INSURED IS EMPLOYED AND COVERED BY EMPLOYER HEALTH PLAN

TELEPHONE NO.

9 OTHER HEALTH INSURANCE COVERAGE (ENTER NAME OF POLICYHOLDER AND PLAN NAME AND ADDRESS AND POLICY OR MEDICAL ASSISTANCE NUMBER)

10 WAS CONDITION RELATED TO:

A PATIENT'S EMPLOYMENT — YES ☐ ☐ NO

B ACCIDENT — AUTO ☐ ☐ OTHER

11 INSURED'S ADDRESS (STREET, CITY, STATE, ZIP CODE)

TELEPHONE NO.

11 a CHAMPUS SPONSOR'S STATUS — ☐ ACTIVE DUTY ☐ DECEASED ☐ RETIRED — BRANCH OF SERVICE

12 PATIENT'S OR AUTHORIZED PERSON'S SIGNATURE (READ BACK BEFORE SIGNING)
I AUTHORIZE THE RELEASE OF ANY MEDICAL INFORMATION NECESSARY TO PROCESS THIS CLAIM. I ALSO REQUEST PAYMENT OF GOVERNMENT BENEFITS EITHER TO MYSELF OR TO THE PARTY WHO ACCEPTS ASSIGNMENT BELOW.

SIGNED DATE

13 I AUTHORIZE PAYMENT OF MEDICAL BENEFITS TO UNDERSIGNED PHYSICIAN OR SUPPLIER FOR SERVICE DESCRIBED BELOW

SIGNED (INSURED OR AUTHORIZED PERSON)

PHYSICIAN OR SUPPLIER INFORMATION

14 DATE OF ◀ ILLNESS (FIRST SYMPTOM) OR INJURY (ACCIDENT) OR PREGNANCY (LMP)

15 DATE FIRST CONSULTED YOU FOR THIS CONDITION

16 IF PATIENT HAS HAD SAME OR SIMILAR ILLNESS OR INJURY GIVE DATES

16 a IF EMERGENCY CHECK HERE ☐

17 DATE PATIENT ABLE TO RETURN TO WORK

18 DATES OF TOTAL DISABILITY — FROM THROUGH

DATES OF PARTIAL DISABILITY — FROM THROUGH

19 NAME OF REFERRING PHYSICIAN OR OTHER SOURCE (e.g. PUBLIC HEALTH AGENCY)

20 FOR SERVICES RELATED TO HOSPITALIZATION GIVE HOSPITALIZATION DATES — ADMITTED DISCHARGED

21 NAME AND ADDRESS OF FACILITY WHERE SERVICES RENDERED (IF OTHER THAN HOME OR OFFICE)

22 WAS LABORATORY WORK PERFORMED OUTSIDE YOUR OFFICE? — YES ☐ ☐ NO CHARGES

23 A DIAGNOSIS OR NATURE OF ILLNESS OR INJURY. RELATE DIAGNOSIS TO PROCEDURE IN COLUMN D BY REFERENCE NUMBERS 1, 2, 3, ETC. OR DX CODE

1

2

3

4

B EPSDT — YES ☐ ☐ NO
FAMILY PLANNING — YES ☐ ☐ NO

PRIOR AUTHORIZATION NO.

24 A DATE OF SERVICE FROM TO	B* PLACE OF SERVICE	C FULLY DESCRIBE PROCEDURES, MEDICAL SERVICES OR SUPPLIES FURNISHED FOR EACH DATE GIVEN — PROCEDURE CODE (IDENTIFY)	(EXPLAIN UNUSUAL SERVICES OR CIRCUMSTANCES)	D DIAGNOSIS CODE	E CHARGES	F DAYS OR UNITS	G* T.O.S.	H LEAVE BLANK

25 SIGNATURE OF PHYSICIAN OR SUPPLIER (INCLUDING DEGREE(S) OR CREDENTIALS) (I CERTIFY THAT THE STATEMENTS ON THE REVERSE APPLY TO THIS BILL AND ARE MADE A PART THEREOF)

DATE

26 ACCEPT ASSIGNMENT (GOVERNMENT CLAIMS ONLY) (SEE BACK) — YES ☐ ☐ NO

27 TOTAL CHARGE

28 AMOUNT PAID

29 BALANCE DUE

30 YOUR SOCIAL SECURITY NO.

31 PHYSICIAN'S, SUPPLIER'S, AND/OR GROUP NAME, ADDRESS, ZIP CODE AND TELEPHONE NO.

I.D. NO.

32 YOUR PATIENT'S ACCOUNT NO.

33 YOUR EMPLOYER I.D. NO.

* PLACE OF SERVICE AND TYPE OF SERVICE (T.O.S.) CODES ON THE BACK
REMARKS

APPROVED BY AMA COUNCIL ON MEDICAL SERVICE 6/83

Form HCFA-1500 (C-2) (1-84) Form OWCP-1500
Form CHAMPUS-501 Form RRB-1500

CHAPTER 2
Medical Considerations

Physicians and clinic staff are accustomed to dealing with a wide variety of patients and their problems. However, certain common problems encountered in providing care for the elderly can be remedied by some of the following recommendations.

Special Services

The practice can offer specialized services for the elderly and can either charge for these new programs or offer them at no cost. Some programs to consider include the following.

Options for the Hearing Impaired. An estimated 17 million Americans suffer from hearing loss, many of whom are over 65. This is a devastating loss because it impairs communication and can lead to frustration, embarrassment and withdrawal. Because they may be embarrassed and uncomfortable with the idea, many patients are reluctant to use a hearing aid. Physicians should encourage their older patients with hearing impairments to see an audiologist. It is important for the physician to know what options are available to sufficiently prepare a patient to see a hearing specialist. Some points which can be stressed are:

- Hearing aids will not help everyone.

- Lives can be changed once a level of hearing is re-established. It is better to hear and participate with a hearing aid than to withdraw and isolate oneself without one.

- Hearing aids are not covered by Medicare and can cost several hundred dollars or more per aid.

- Physicians may choose to monitor and encourage use of the hearing devices.

The following describes some of the most popular hearing aid devices.

- Body-type hearing aids are worn in a pocket or on a belt with a cord leading up to the ear. These are the most powerful type of hearing aids. Many people object to body-type hearing aids because they are so visible.

- Behind-the-ear hearing aids are shaped like a half-moon and fit behind the ear with a small, clear tube leading to the earmold.

- All-in-the-ear types of hearing aids fit totally in the earmold. These are the most popular aids.

- Canal hearing aids are the smallest aids available. There are no earmolds and they fit directly into an ear canal.

- A "listen box" is a box-type device which looks like a small portable transistor radio with earphones. The patient can easily carry this type of hearing device for conversation or for use at home to watch television. It is a good idea to have one of these available in the office so the medical staff can communicate more clearly with a patient.

- Flashers, which signal to a patient by the flashing of a light, are available for alarm clocks, door bells and telephones. These devices are hooked to a lamp that will flash on and off to alert the hearing impaired person when the alarm clock is sounding or the doorbell or phone is ringing.

- Other telephone aids include volume controls and small amplifiers for the telephone ear piece. Call the phone company for details.

Hearing screenings and evaluations can be performed in a physician's office by providing a space for an audiologist on an as-needed basis. This service can be used by both the older and younger patients of the practice. Medicare will reimburse for a hearing evaluation.

Incontinence Clinic. Urinary incontinence affects 15 to 30 percent of the elderly in the community and at least half of all nursing home residents. Of the 10 million Americans with this condition, 50 percent have had no evaluation or treatment. There is a persistent myth that urinary incontinence is a normal consequence of aging. It has been found that urinary incontinence does not result directly from aging, but that age-related changes in the urinary tract may predispose some older adults to this condition. Physicians, working in conjunction with urologists, may address the incontinence issue in the practice setting by offering clinics on such topics as bladder training, pelvic muscle exercises and biofeedback.

Medication Monitoring. Assuring the accurate and timely administration of dosages of medications can be difficult when working with frail, older adults. Some suggestions to prevent multiple or insufficient dosages are:

- Ask your drug representative for a supply of pill boxes which have one compartment for each day of the week and separate sections for different times of the day. With some training, a frail adult may learn to take accurate dosages by using the pill box properly.

- Prepare a large print, easy to read label to tape over the existing label. For example: TAKE ONE PILL AT BEDTIME.

- Create a list of which medications are to be taken. Include the time and the amount to be taken.

A family member, a neighbor or a volunteer can be assigned to coordinate medications for older people. The staff of home health care agencies can also help with medication monitoring. If the patient continues to misuse medications, an assisted living facility may be an appropriate alternative to independent living. In an assisted living facility, medications are administered by staff to ensure proper usage.

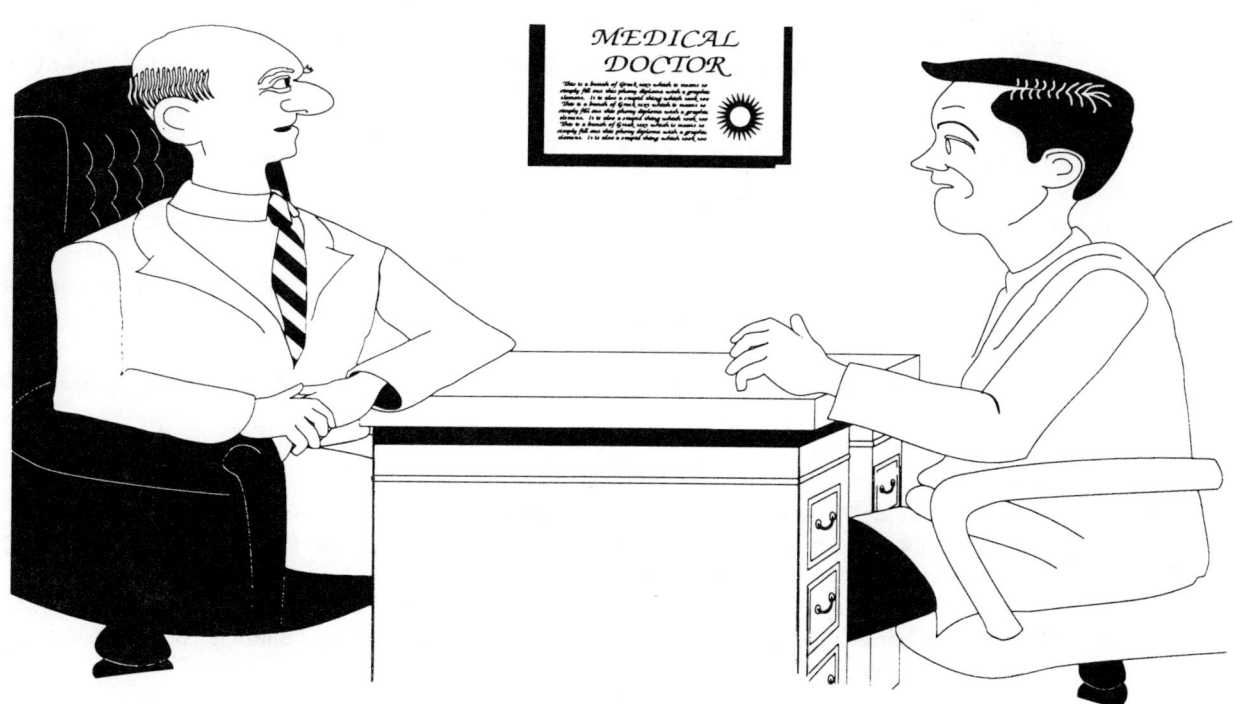

"Doc, I think I'm experiencing side-effects from that placebo you prescribed for me."

Medical Equipment and Supplies

Special considerations need to be taken with older patients to increase their level of comfort. Frequently, small adjustments in existing or new equipment can achieve this goal. Many times the small changes are inexpensive, but they offer significant improvements in the quality of the care received. The following are some suggestions for the purchase of new equipment and some ideas for adjusting existing equipment with the geriatric patient in mind.

Supplies.
- Use plastic speculums instead of metal. Metal can further irritate existing urinary tract infections in older women. It is also important to have smaller-sized speculums available.

- Stock adult disposable diapers in case of accidents.

- If the office gowns are thin and easy to see through, give the patient two gowns. Show the patient how to put one gown on back to front and the other on front to back so all of their body is covered.

- Oxygen should be available for older patients who have breathing difficulties.

- A mist nebulizer should be available for people who have respiratory distress.

- An oximeter, a device for measuring oxygen content in the blood, is a basic piece of equipment needed when working with the elderly.

- Have bowel and gall bladder prep kits available in the office to save patients an extra trip to the hospital before scheduled tests.

Equipment.
- A wheelchair can be very useful to have in a clinic. It can help get the patient to the exam room from the waiting room if there is an emergency or even if the patient just has difficulty walking and needs help.

- Have a stretcher available which can collapse to floor level should a patient fall or have a seizure while in the office.

- Purchase a "listen box" which can be used by a hearing impaired patient to amplify sound when communicating with staff at the office. (See "Options for the Hearing Impaired," presented earlier in this chapter, for further explanation of a listen box.)

X-ray Equipment.
- A table pad reduces discomfort for patients receiving x-rays.

- Provide a step stool to help patients on and off the x-ray table.

- If a patient must maintain a set position for an x-ray for an extended period of time, an IV pole can be used to support the patient's arms.

- A 4-way float top x-ray table can be an expensive but valuable addition to existing equipment. This table top allows the x-ray technician to slide the table top instead of pulling and pushing the patient.

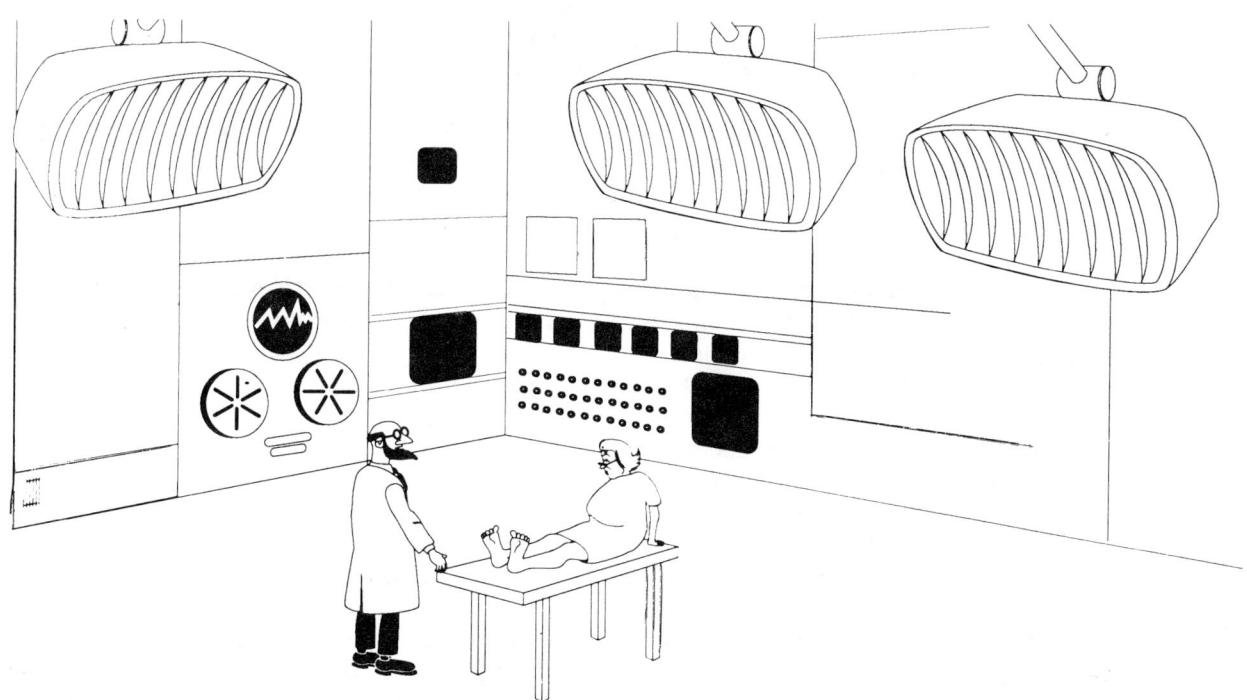

"So, Mrs. Crimfister, I understand we have an owie on our little toe."

Medical Records

Older adults visit the physician's office more frequently than younger patients. Consequently, their medical records are usually larger. Three areas of the medical record—demographics, psycho/social and a flow chart—can be added or modified to save time by pinpointing often needed information within the chart more efficiently.

Demographics. Often insurance information is kept separate from the chart. The addition of a demographic and insurance section to the medical record can save time when making referrals or follow-up phone calls.

Psycho/Social. A baseline psycho/social history, taken as part of the initial physical, will give the clinician additional information to make medical decisions. The psycho/social history should detail the patient's support system, housing and financial situation. Many assessment tools are available to assess a patient's level of functioning. Consider adding a self-administered assessment instrument as a part of the intake procedure. Contact CRAHCA for available assessment tools.

Flow Sheet. A case management flow sheet can provide information at a glance regarding a patient's status and needs over time. (See CHAPTER 4—Referrals and Exhibit 4 on page 22.) The flow sheet can be especially helpful in large, busy practices because it supports communication among providers and promotes continuity of care.

A case management flow sheet can take the place of a problem list and is more comprehensive. The case management flow sheet should be placed at the front of the record to provide the following information at a glance:
— Patient's name
— Patient's birthday
— Notes regarding psycho/social information
— Problems the patient is experiencing
— Severity level of problems
— Names of other physicians who have seen the patient
— A view of the patient's medical history over an eight-visit span

To use the flow sheet, complete the demographic information at the top of the document prior to the patient's first encounter. For each encounter, indicate the date and type of encounter and the current problem. A code, indicating the provider's evaluation of the patient's current status, should be assigned to each problem.

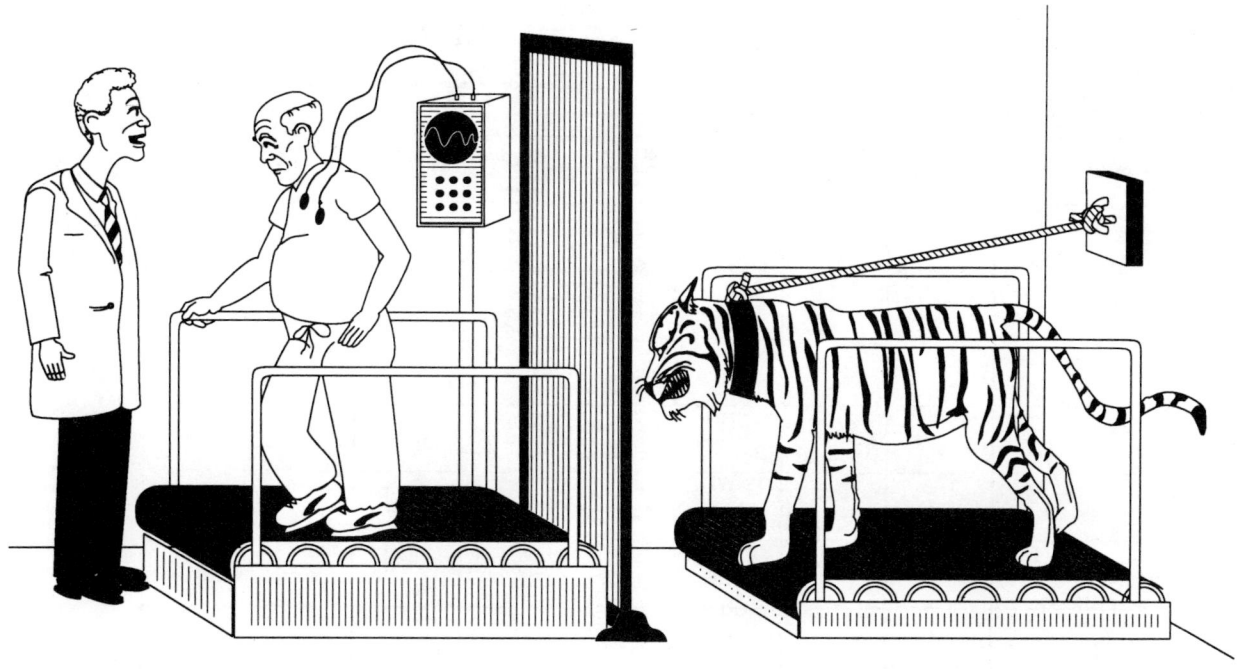

"We have recently perfected a technique that guarantees you'll reach maximum heart rate."

Exhibit 4

CASE MANAGEMENT FLOW SHEET

NAME_____
Date of Birth_____

PATIENT PROFILE
Important individual factors (e.g. housing, living arrangements, care giver, etc.)
_____
_____
_____

Status Codes:

A = No problem requiring action or problem resolved
B = Stable, no action or change in action required
C = Minor problem or change in status requiring action
D = Serious problem or change in status requiring action
E = Admit to hospital
F = Other

(Circled codes also have narrative notes in chart)

Date: PROBLEM	Clinic Cnfrnce H.Visit	Clinic Cnfrnce H.Visit	Clinic Cnfrnce H.Visit	Clinic Cnfrnce H.Visit	Clinic Cnfrnce H.Visit	Clinic Cnfrnce H.Visit	Clinic Cnfrnce H.Visit	Clinic Cnfrnce H.Visit

Copyright © GeriMed of America, Inc., 1989
All Rights Reserved

CHAPTER 3
Patient Education

Patient education in medical care is a fairly new concept. Many older people, as well as some younger ones, hesitate to ask questions regarding their health care. If the physician and staff take time to educate and teach patients about their conditions, they will be more apt to ask questions and in turn better able to care for themselves.

Pamphlets, handouts and classes are all effective means of communicating with patients. By increasing communication to patients, they will be better informed and more apt to return to the physician who goes that extra mile to provide quality, well-rounded care.

Pamphlets

Pamphlets can be used to further explain a medical condition to a patient. For example, if a patient has osteoporosis, the physician can explain the condition and then hand the patient a pamphlet on the subject to take home and read. This can minimize the time the physician spends with the patient and help answer questions by filling in gaps once the patient is home.

If possible, have a brochure rack in the entryway or waiting area. There are many brochures geared towards the 65 and over population. A good source of information for brochures for older people is the American Association of Retired Persons (AARP), 1901 K Street N.W., Washington D.C. 20049.

Handouts

Handouts with specially written instructions or procedures can be a helpful tool. Many associations, including pharmaceutical companies, provide literature on particular medical topics. Make sure the handouts are easy to read and understand. If possible, use illustrations.

The following are some suggested topics for handouts:
- Low sodium diets
- Low fat diets
- Bland diets
- Diabetic diets
- Low cholesterol diets
- Diarrhea diets
- Upper GI (Gastrointestinal)
- Barium Enema
- Gallbladder series
- MRI (Magnetic Radiographic Imaging)
- EMG (Electromyography)
- CT (Computed Tomography) Scan/Bone Scan
- Medication Monitoring

Educational Classes

Educational classes can be taught by either a staff member or a community professional. The waiting room (before or after patient hours), an exam room or a room at a nearby hospital can serve adequately for educational classes. Classes should be held periodically to educate the current patient base or to market to new patients.

Some suggested subjects are:
- Arthritis self-help
- Living with osteoporosis
- Dealing with Medicare billing
- Selecting supplemental insurance
- Types of diets
- Tricks to weight loss
- Evaluating your health
- Mammography and breast self-exam

(See CHAPTER VI - Marketing for further information.)

Tips for Healthy Living Booklet

A booklet called *Tips for Healthy Living* was designed by GeriMed of America to give patients very basic information on health care. Topics in the booklet include:
- Exercise and Nutrition
- Foot Care
- Healthy Sleep
- Skin Care
- Using Medications Safely
- Over the Counter Drug Information

This type of booklet is an excellent handout to give to new patients and is also helpful as a marketing tool. (See Exhibit 5 on page 27 for a sample page from the *Tips for Healthy Living* booklet.)

Patient Handbook

A model patient handbook was designed by GeriMed of America to encourage patients to take an active role in their health care and to provide information about their physician's office. The handbook is given to the patient during his or her first visit to the physician's office. The patient handbook is beneficial to both the patient and the physician as long as they both participate. The office and medical staff might need to remind and encourage patients to use the handbook. It is a new concept and it may take time for patients to adjust to it.

A typical handbook may include sections on:
- How the office works (hours, phone numbers, after hours procedures)
- Who the staff members are and what they do
- Transportation to and from the physician's office
- Medicare and bills
- Blank pages for notes from the physician
- Blank pages for questions to ask the physician
- Blood pressure and weight monitors
- Current medication list

The patient handbook is beneficial to the patient because:

- It helps them take an active role in their health care.

- By providing space to write down thoughts, opinions and questions, it serves as a reminder so the patient can discuss his/her health care with the physician.

- It better educates the patients on health care in general and helps them to monitor their own health care.

The handbook is beneficial to the physician because:

- It provides a space for the patient to keep track of current medications which should be checked by the physician at each visit.

- It saves the physician and staff time because it gives preliminary explanations of billing statements, office procedures, health care information and more.

(For some sample pages from a patient handbook, please see Exhibit 6 on pages 28 through 30.)

Healthy Lifestyle Approaches Booklet

The Duluth Clinic, Limited, in Minnesota has developed a booklet, *Healthy Lifestyle Approaches* with support from the W. K. Kellogg Foundation in conjunction with CRAHCA. This booklet was designed to encourage patients to take a look at their lifestyles and identify areas for self-improvement. Included in this booklet are tips on various health-related topics. Patients are encouraged to share the information in the booklet with their physicians.

Topics included in this booklet include:
- Personal History
- Physical Health History
- Personal Medication Record
- Managing Medications
- Reducing Cancer Risk
- Reducing Cardiac Problems
- General Symptoms
- Sensory Information
- Nutrition Information
- Emotional Well-Being
- Activity Suggestions
- Anxiety/Tension/Stress
- Coping with Depression
- Dealing with Anger
- Problem-Solving Suggestions
- Memory Information
- Daily Living Activities
- Home Environmental Information
- Economic Well-Being

(For sample pages from the *Healthy Lifestyle Approaches* booklet, please see Exhibit 7 on pages 31 and 32.)

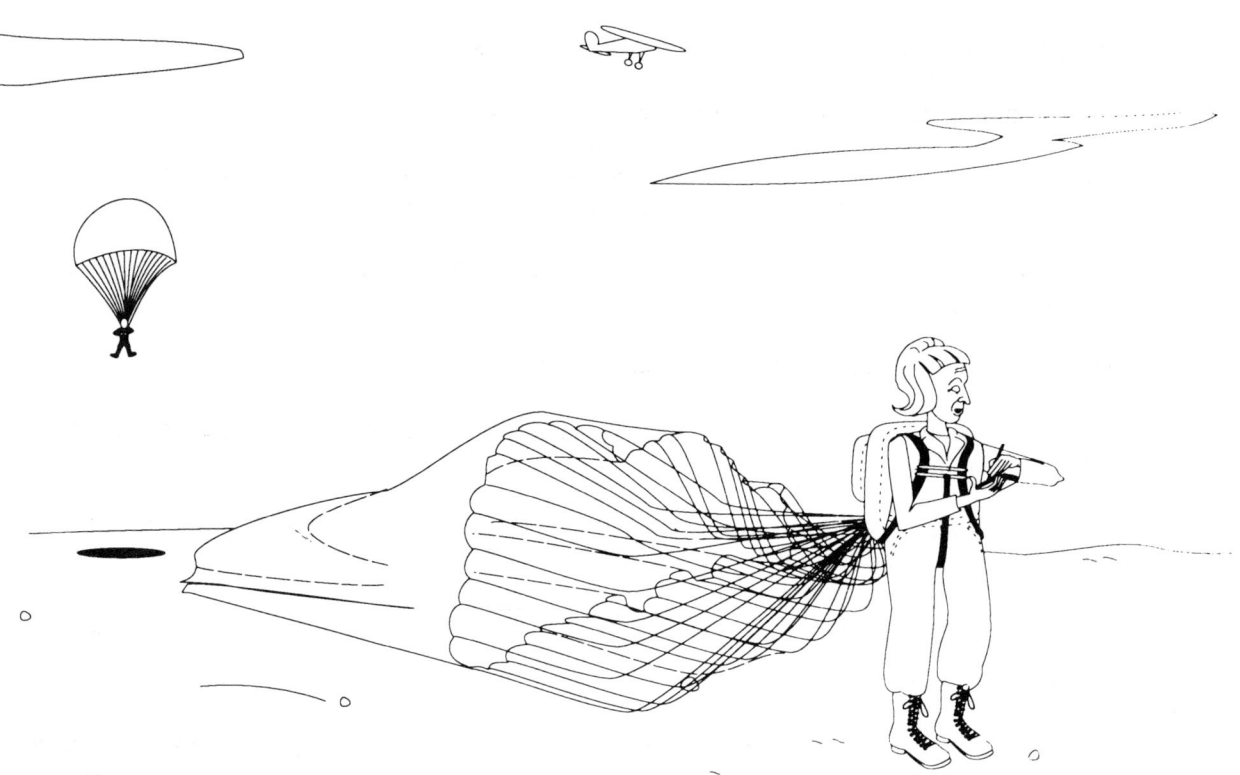

"It's been on my 'to do' list for 25 years, but I finally got THAT out of the way."

Newsletters

Newsletters published by the practice can be a source of information for new and established patients alike. Over and above their obvious use as a marketing tool, newsletters can be used to publicize the latest medical developments and announce upcoming classes and clinics sponsored by the practice. Articles can expand on topics presented in the patient handbook or in a "tips" booklet, or the newest technology aimed toward the senior patient can be announced. A section could also be set aside as a "Patient's Corner," either for questions and answers about subjects of interest or self-help articles written by patients. Newletters should be informative and interesting and should be published on a regular basis.

Exhibit 5

SAMPLE PAGE - TIPS FOR HEALTHY LIVING BOOKLET

USING YOUR MEDICATIONS SAFELY

DO

- Take only the amount of medication your doctor prescribes and follow the dosage and frequency schedule.

- Let your doctor know what medications you are currently taking and any allergies you are aware of.

- Call your doctor if you experience any side effects to the medication you are taking.

- Make it your business to find out from the doctor or pharmacist how your medications work together. This also includes medicine you can buy without a prescription.

DON'T

- Don't stop taking your medication because you feel better. Take them for as long as your doctor told you to.

- Don't keep any old medications that have expired. Many medications lose their effectiveness when they get old.

- Don't mix your medications with alcohol unless your doctor says it is O.K.

- Don't exchange medications with someone else. Take only medications prescribed for you.

- Don't break pills or crush pills without asking your doctor or pharmacist.

Copyright © GenMed of America, Inc., 1989
All Rights Reserved

Exhibit 6
Sample Pages from the Patient Handbook

Appointments and Phone Calls.

APPOINTMENTS AND PHONE CALLS

Appointments

We recommend a scheduled appointment to see our health care staff. When scheduling your appointment, please give a brief description of your concerns. You will be scheduled at a time that is convenient for you.

Call - 586-8600, Monday through Friday 8:30 A.M. - 5:00 P.M.

We encourage new patients to have a comprehensive physical exam. This exam enables the physician to understand your medical history and current medical needs. These appointments are usually scheduled for approximately two hours.

We realize that from time to time you need to cancel an appointment. We would appreciate at least 24-hours' notice. When you cancel, we suggest you reschedule your appointment.

Phone Calls

Our doctor is happy to speak to you on the telephone. Due to his busy schedule, morning calls will be returned by the end of the morning. Your afternoon call will be returned at the end of the day. Please let us know if other arrangements for returning your calls need to be made.

If you call with an emergency, the doctor or nurse will be contacted immediately to help you. If you need to be seen by our doctor, arrangements will be made. If, however, this is an extreme emergency, call the paramedics at 911.

When you need a prescription drug refilled, call the pharmacy and request a refill. The pharmacist will then call your physician. Call early in the day so the pharmacist can refill the medication in one day. We recommend you call your pharmacist before your medication runs out.

Copyright © GeriMed of America, Inc., 1989
All Rights Reserved

Exhibit 6
Sample Pages from the Patient Handbook (continued)

Your Medication List.

YOUR MEDICATION LIST

This is where you can keep a record of your current medication, the dosage, frequency and date started. There is also a column to indicate additional comments regarding your medications. In order to keep your list up to date, draw a line through the medications that get discontinued.

Medications	What for?	Dosage (How Much)	Frequency (How Often)	Date Started	Additional Comments
Example					
1. Lasix	Blood Pressure	2 tablets	3 × per day	3/1/89	Best to take after meals
2.					
3.					
4.					
5.					
6.					
7.					
8.					

Copyright © GeriMed of America, Inc., 1989
All Rights Reserved

Exhibit 6
Sample Pages from the Patient Handbook (continued)

Questions to Ask.
We are sure you will agree that it is important for you to understand the issues surrounding your health care. That is why we welcome your questions and even provide a space for you to jot them down. You can write them down when you think of a question whether you are in the clinic or even at home.

We will be happy to take the time to answer your questions about your health needs. Please take an active part in your health care and ask questions.

We have provided you with a sample question and answer below. Please feel free to use it as a guide for your own questions.

Sample Question *Date: 3-1-89*

What is blood pressure and what do the top and bottom numbers mean?

Sample Answer *Date: 3-1-89*

Blood pressure is the measurement of the force of blood against the artery walls. The bottom number is the blood's pressure during the relaxation part in between heartbeats. The top number is the pressure of the blood against the walls of the arteries during the actual beat of the heart.

Exhibit 7
Sample Pages from the *Healthy Lifestyles Approaches* Booklet

Emotional Well-Being.

Do you have someone you confide in? _____ Yes _____ No

Describe a typical day: _____
_____
_____

List the activities in which you participate:

_____   _____
_____   _____
_____   _____

What do you do to relax?
_____
_____
_____
_____

How often do you receive visits from or visit someone in a week? _____

How many telephone calls do you make or receive in a week? _____

Are you satisfied with the amount of social contact you have?

_____ Yes   _____ No

Exhibit 7
Sample Pages from the *Healthy Lifestyles Approaches* Booklet (continued)

Sensory.

<u>VISION</u>

I CAN _____ See Newsprint   _____ Headlines

_____ Obstacles In My Path   _____ Tell Light From Dark

_____ Not See

To make the most of your vision:

1. Put items in the same place
2. Use bright colors
3. Ask a friend to help you with color selection or matching colors
4. Place items where you can see them
5. Use magnifying devices

For help with vision:

See your physician for a medical evaluation

Contact: Minnesota State Services for the Blind and Visually Handicapped/Elder Options
723-4600

<u>HEARING</u>

I CAN _____ Hear without having the person raise their voice both with one person or in groups

_____ Hear with one person but have difficulty in groups

_____ Hear with a firm clear volume, face-to-face

_____ Not hear

To make the most of your hearing:

1. Have the speaker face you
2. Ask the speaker to <u>rephrase</u> unclear messages
3. Ask the speaker to speak slower, enunciate clearly, and lower their voice
4. Eliminate background noise
5. Make sure you can see the speaker's mouth
6. Encourage the speaker to use gestures

For help with hearing:

See you physician for a medical evaluation

Contact: The Regional Service Center for Hearing Impaired

TDD: 723-4961   VOICE: 723-4962

<u>IF A HEARING AID IS PRESCRIBED - WEAR IT!</u>

CHAPTER 4
Referrals

There are many services throughout the country which are dedicated to helping older people and their families. But often, assessing patient needs and finding the appropriate service can be time consuming. If the physician feels that his patients need more than he or she can provide, case management services can be an answer. As defined in *The Encyclopedia of Social Work,* "Case management is an approach to service delivery that attempts to ensure that clients with complex problems and disabilities receive all the services they need in a timely and appropriate fashion." Case management services parallel the medical responsibilities of the physician and provide the patient with much needed services. According to Robert A. Berenson in an article he wrote for *Business and Health,* (July/August 1985) "... making physicians medical managers, as in case management, means they are responsible for providing all primary health care services, as well as coordinating and approving the provision of other health care, including specialty care and hospitalization." Case managers are well versed on community services and can coordinate those services to meet the needs of their clients.

A case manager can be hired by a large practice, or an existing staff member can be designated to become familiar with local services and agencies. Also, social workers are often available in the community who will provide case management services on a sliding scale or a fee for service basis. (For more information on case management, refer to CRAHCA's *Case Management Manual.*)

If patients do not need extensive case management referrals, physicians can become familiar with the types of programs offered and the agencies which provide services. Help is available in the areas of activities of daily living (ADLs), housing, social service, mental health, finance, law, emergency, abuse and medicine. Below are programs available for the elderly and some typical agencies which may be available in a community. (See Appendix 2 for names and addresses of local referral agencies.)

Activities of Daily Living (ADLs)

Activities of Daily Living (ADLs) are those normal daily activities such as dressing and undressing, grooming, feeding oneself, cooking and toileting which determine a person's level of independence. Physicians and other medical personnel can become aware of the patient's living conditions by asking questions. "Is the patient losing weight due to inadequate eating habits?" "Are family members burned out from caring for their loved one?" "Does the patient need help in his or her home with meals, housecleaning or yardwork?" "Can the patient still function in his or her own home?" Help is available through services such as those outlined below.

Adult Day Care. Adult day care centers provide a place where physically or psychologically impaired people go during the day for socialization, recreational activities and lunch. They are geared toward keeping the frail elderly independent in the community and providing respite to families. Adult day care centers vary in terms of programs offered. Some centers are geared toward social activities while others have a medical component as well. Adult day care centers are often managed by hospitals. Contact The National Institute on Adult Day Care for further information.

Alzheimer's Assistance. Programs are available for patients and families of those afflicted with Alzheimer's disease. These programs include Alzheimer's adult day care programs, respite care in the home by specially trained companions, nursing homes with special Alzheimer's wings, family support groups and more. Call the National Alzheimer's Association or your local chapter for more information regarding services in specific areas.

Family Support Networks. Adult children often juggle their lives to help their parents, even though there are many services to help older people. The caretakers often need support and education to help understand and accommodate their parents' needs. Classes and support groups are available on a variety of subjects such as adult children of aging parents and helping families understand Alzheimer's. For more information contact the Area Agency on Aging or a local college or university.

Home Delivered Meals. Some elderly are not able to prepare a nutritional meal for themselves. Either after an illness, on a temporary basis or on a permanent basis, meals can be brought into the home by volunteers for no cost or on a donation basis. Many different agencies across the country provide home delivered meals. Call the Area Agency on Aging for more information.

Homemakers. The elderly often need help with the basic necessities of running a home. Homemakers are people who are paid either through an agency or privately to help people clean their homes, cook meals or just be companions. Call a national home health care agency or the Area Agency on Aging to obtain information about local homemaker services.

Hospice. Terminally ill patients may want to die at home or in a homelike environment. Hospice (meaning "terminally ill") care was developed to provide a comfortable environment for the dying. Hospice care, including both medical and psycho/social care, can be provided in a patient's home or in a group facility. Medicare covers some costs of hospice care. Call the National Hospice Organization or the Hospice Education Institute for more information on local hospice care.

Respite Care - In Home. The term "respite" means a temporary intermission. Agencies, as well as private pay workers, are available to provide respite for families who are caring for older, frail adults. A person will come in and stay with the older adult for a period of time ranging from an hour to several weeks while the caretaker is relieved of duties. Contact the National Association for Home Care for further information.

Respite Care - Outside Home. Many facilities offer a room to an older person for a few days to a few weeks while his/her caretakers are out of town. These facilities include assisted living facilities and nursing homes. Look in the Yellow Pages under "Senior Citizen Services" or "Nursing Homes" for names of facilities which might offer this service or contact the American Association of Homes for the Aging.

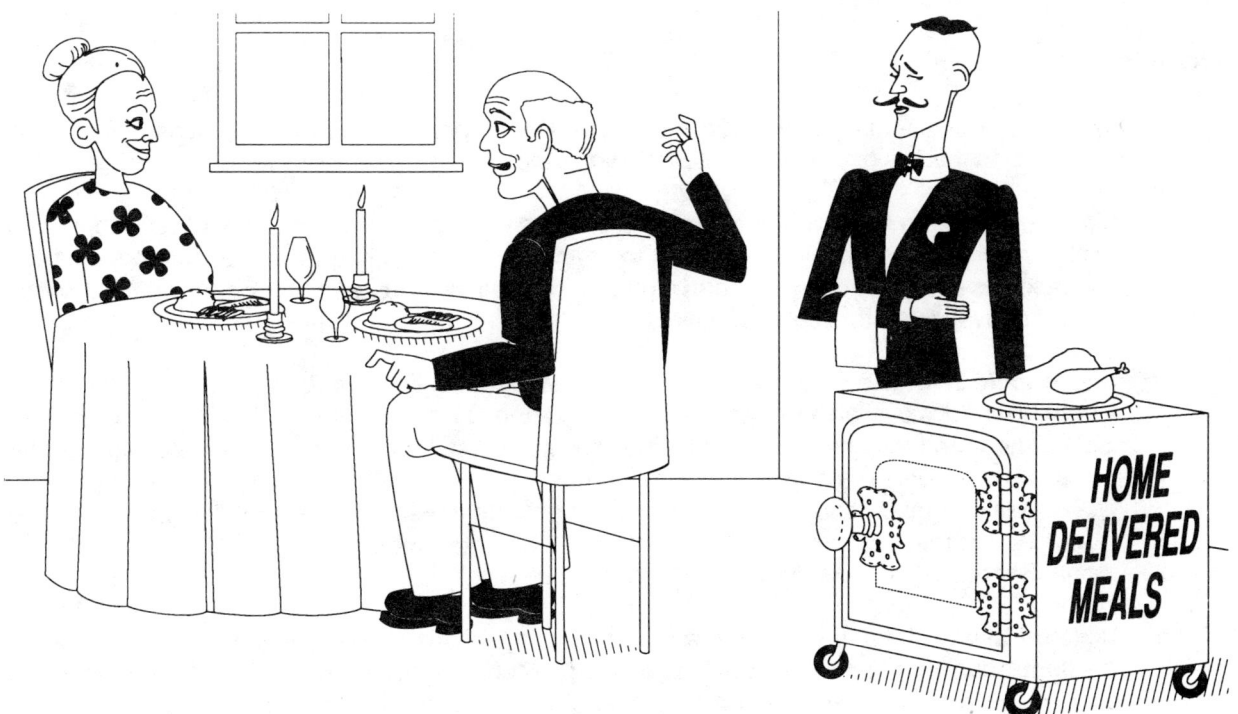

"He says the fancy door leads down to the wine cellar."

Senior Companions. Senior Companions are older people who are paid a stipend for visiting older, more frail persons on a weekly basis. Companions provide support and friendship to more isolated seniors. Contact the local Area Agency on Aging for additional information.

Transportation. Many older people no longer drive for a variety of reasons. Lack of transportation services is a major concern. Some agencies offer rides to seniors on a fee-for-service or donation basis to restricted services. For example, it may be easier to get a ride to a physician's office but more difficult to get to a drugstore. Contact the Area Agency on Aging for more resource information regarding transportation or look in the Yellow Pages under "Senior Services - Transportation."

Meal Sites - Outside Home. Usually senior centers provide an area where older people can eat a well-balanced lunch in a group setting five times per week. The seniors are asked to make a donation for their meals. Contact local senior centers, churches, synagogues or the Area Agency on Aging for available sites.

Housing

A physician might feel a patient is placing himself in danger by living alone. Or a patient may tell the physician that it is getting too difficult for him to care for his Alzheimer's wife in their large home.

It is very difficult to leave a home regardless of the reasons. Although many older people can continue to live in their homes, many opt to change their living situations to accommodate their decreased level of functioning. Others bring services into their homes so they can remain at home. Below are available housing alternatives.

Independent Living. People who are functionally independent all or most of the time have a variety of living situations available to them and a broad range of housing options. For more information, contact the American Association of Homes for the Aging. Independent living facilities include:
— Private home or condominium
— Age integrated and age segregated apartments, such as retirement living facilities
— Government apartments, both subsidized and non-subsidized
— Shared housing for financial reasons

Assisted Living. People who need assistance with activities of daily living and/or medication monitoring can live in an assisted living facility. They offer more services than independent living facilities, but less than nursing home care. Assisted living facilities include:
— Board and care homes or small homes which offer a bedroom and shared common living areas
— Apartment-style facilities that offer private apartments with all services included
— Shared living with another person for supportive help

Call the American Association of Homes for the Aging for more information on local assisted living facilities.

Nursing Homes. Nursing homes provide a living environment for people requiring 24-hour care and daily medical, nursing, psycho/social and rehabilitative services. Contact the American Association of Homes for the Aging or the state ombudsman office for information on nursing homes and how to choose one.

Housing services available for persons choosing to remain in their own homes may include the following.

Housecleaning/Homemaker Assistance. Housecleaning and Homemaker services are available for those who wish to stay in their own home but might not be able to perform such tasks as vacuuming, laundering, shopping and cooking. These services can be hired for one hour a week to a few hours a day and more. A worker may come into the home and clean or make lunch and prepare the evening meal in advance so the older person just has to warm it up at mealtime. This can be a very flexible service geared to meet the individual needs of the older person. Some people may be eligible to receive assistance through social service agencies. Other agencies to contact are the American Federation of Home Health and the National Association of Home Care.

Utility Assistance. Most states offer assistance with utility bills in rebate form to eligible older people on limited incomes. Call the state or county Social Services Department or the local Public Service Company for more details.

Weatherization. Home weatherization services are often free to those who are in need of insulation for their homes and apartments. Often there are no income eligibility requirements. Services are usually offered by counties or through a service organization of the Area Agency on Aging.

Yardwork Assistance. Yardwork assistance can be obtained for those who want to stay in their homes and cannot manage the upkeep of a yard. Often school programs sponsor groups of students who volunteer their time, or the service can be purchased from local lawn care companies which may offer senior discounts.

Grocery Delivery Services. Many grocery stores offer free delivery service for the home bound. The staff may be paid by the store or a volunteer delivery service may be used. Grocery stores or retirement housing complexes may even offer free transportation to and from the grocery store. Contact local grocery stores to inquire about these services.

Social

Ongoing social contact is a vital part of combating the loneliness and depression that can result from the losses that occur as one ages. People continue to grow and stay more alert by maintaining active social lives. The social opportunities described below can assist people who live alone and do not see many people but feel the need for more contact.

Congregate Meal Programs. These programs offer well-balanced meals in a group setting. Some areas even provide free transportation to the sites. They are usually located in senior centers, churches and synagogues or contact the Area Agency on Aging for local meal sites.

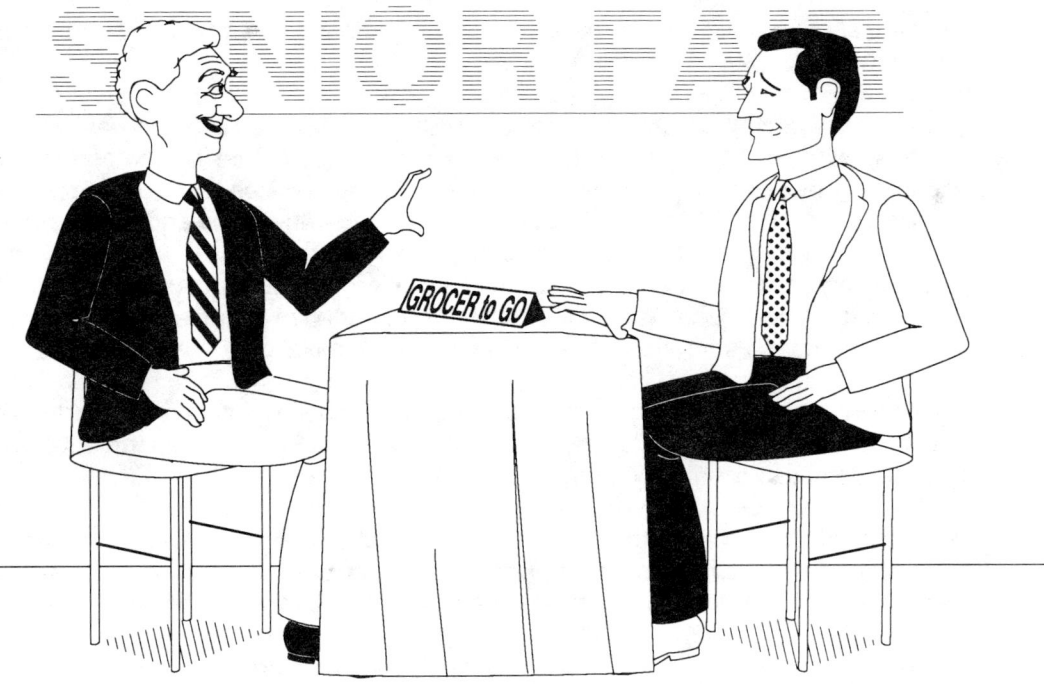

"Now before I hire your grocery delivery service I'll have to give you a little test on the proper wrist action to deploy while squeezing a melon."

Employment Opportunities. Some states offer specialized services for older people seeking job opportunities. Contact the Area Agency on Aging or the State Employment Office for details.

Senior Centers/Community Centers. Many communities have centers with programs specifically for older people. These centers offer a variety of programs that range from overnight trips to card groups. Many centers offer schedules of programs to fit a variety of interests. The Area Agency on Aging can assist with finding a center nearby. Also look in the Yellow Pages under "Senior Citizen Services."

Telephone Reassurance Check. Usually volunteers donate time to call a frail or at-risk person at the same time every day to check in and offer support and reassurance. If no one answers the phone, a contact person is called to check on the older person. If a contact person cannot be reached, the police are called to investigate. This service may be sponsored by the Volunteers of America or contact the Area Agency on Aging.

Volunteer Opportunities. Many opportunities are available for volunteers. These opportunities can be learning experiences offering both enrichment and satisfaction for those donating their time. Contact the Volunteers of America, the Retired Senior Volunteer Program (RSVP) or a favorite charity for further information.

Mental Health

Has a patient come to the office crying and upset over the death of a spouse even though it has been over a year since the death? Has a patient ever expressed a desire to end his or her life? Several options are available to help physicians with patients who are struggling with a mental health problem.

Mental Health Centers. These centers provide mental health services within communities. They often have staff social workers and psychologists who are skilled in serving the older population. Many centers offer services at no cost or on a sliding-fee-scale basis. Contact the National Institute for Mental Health for the name of a local center.

Peer Counselor. Peer counseling programs train older people to listen, empathize and provide information to other, more frail, older people. The peer counselors are usually continually trained by mental health professionals and volunteer their time for this program. Contact the Area Agency on Aging for more information.

Psychologist/Psychiatrist. Psychologists and psychiatrists are trained to work with older people and their problems. Some psychiatric services are paid for under Medicare. These professionals can be found in the Yellow Pages or contact your local hospital to identify an appropriate mental health professional.

Social Workers. Social workers perform a variety of tasks, including counseling, case management, information and referral and more. Some social workers are trained in gerontology and can assist older people seeking help. Some community agencies offer social work or case management services at no cost or on a sliding-fee-scale. Contact the National Institute of Mental Health or the Area Agency on Aging for further information on social work services.

Support Groups. Support groups are available to help family members understand and cope with a variety of age-related topics. Groups are also available to aid older people with such problems as diabetes, alcoholism, grief and more. Contact the National Institute on Mental Health or look in the Yellow Pages under the area of need such as "Counseling." Also the Area Agency on Aging is a good source of information on support groups. Newspapers often print a list of local support groups periodically.

Admission to a Psychiatric Hospital. Gero-psych hospitals or gero-psych units of hospitals provide inpatient psychological treatment specifically for people over age 65. Contact a local hospital or look in the Yellow Pages under "Mental Health Services" for more information.

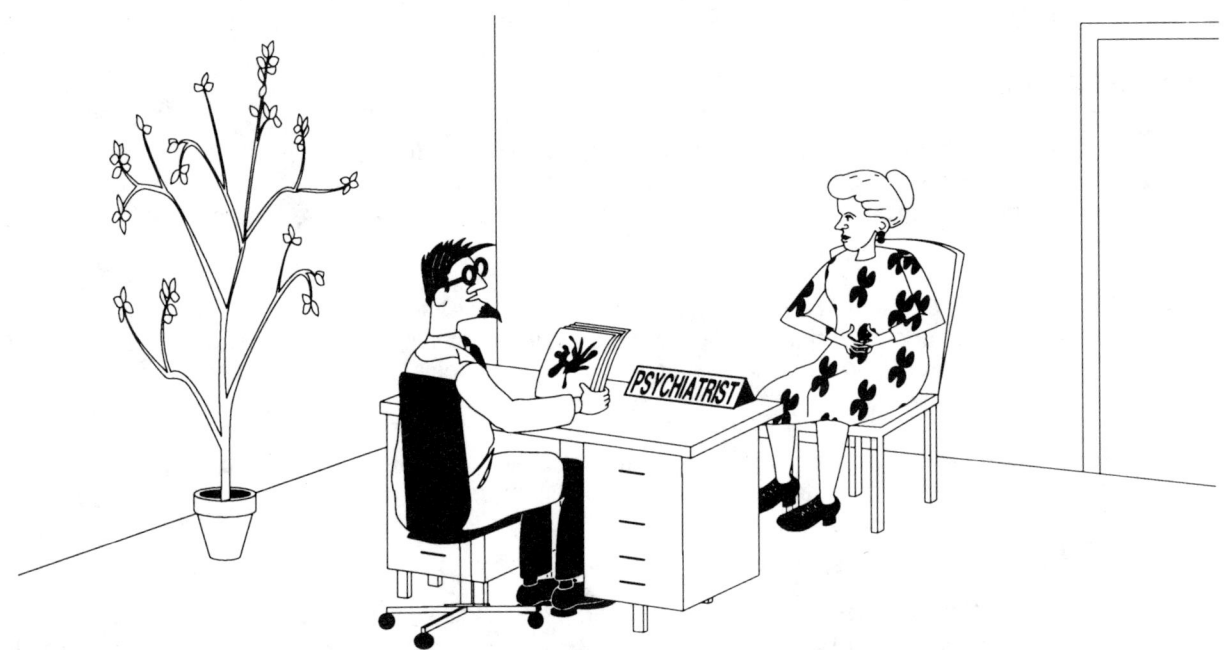

"Now remember there are no right answers in this test. You will, however, be given a final grade."

Financial and Legal Assistance

Financial and legal services are two areas where seniors often need assistance. If they qualify, low income seniors may be able to receive additional income per month and/or be placed on a program which helps with medical bills. Lower cost legal services are also available. The following are some financial and legal resources available for patients who need assistance.

Food Stamps. Food stamps are available for those who are income eligible. Medicaid/Medi-Cal recipients may qualify. Contact a local Social Services office for more information.

Insurance Counseling. An independent insurance counselor can assist patients with selection of an appropriate supplemental policy. This is a relatively new area. Contact the Area Agency on Aging to find out if counseling is available locally.

Legal Assistance. No-cost or low-cost legal help is available for those who are income eligible. Assistance can range from preparation of wills to help with writing and signing contracts. Some universities offer free services. Contact a local law school or the National Senior Citizens Law Center for more information.

Medicaid/Medi-Cal. Medicaid/Medi-Cal programs are funded by state and federal governments and financially assist low income people who meet the requirements by offering extended health care insurance. This program also helps defray the cost of nursing home care. Medicaid eligibility is not based on straight income. Some states offer Medicaid to those who have very high medical bills and are in need of assistance. Contact the Adult Unit of the county Social Service Office for more information.

Medicare. Medicare is a health insurance program offered by the federal government to all American citizens over age 65. Medicare has two parts, A and B. Part A covers inpatient hospital care while Part B assists with physician costs and other services not covered by Part A. (For a more detailed description see CHAPTER 2 under "Billing.") Call the local Social Security office for further information on Medicare eligibility.

Social Security — Supplemental Security Income. The Supplemental Security Income program supplements social security for low income people who are blind, disabled or aged. More information can be obtained by calling the local Social Security office.

Social Security — Old Age Survivors and Disabled Insurance. Most people age 65 and over are eligible to receive Social Security. People who have paid into the system through employment for a certain number of quarter-years are eligible to receive a monthly check from the Social Security System as are their spouses and ex-spouses. Call the local Social Security office for details.

Social Services. Social Services in some states offer financial assistance to low income elderly. Call the county Adult or Aging Unit for qualifying information.

Emergency or Abusive Assistance

Has a patient come in frightened after being mugged? Is the physician concerned that a family member is abusing a patient? Services which can protect elderly people from abusive or emergency situations include the following.

Adult Protective Services. Adult Protective Services offer protection for older people. If mental or physical abuse, neglect or mistreatment is suspected, call the county Social Services Department. An anonymous call can be placed. The department staff are required to act on each complaint.

Crime Victim Assistance. Recently agencies have started programs to aid victims of crime. Some agencies have staff who are sensitive to the needs of older people. These agencies provide support and sometimes minimal financial assistance. Call the county Victims' Assistance program through the police department or contact the Area Agency on Aging.

Emergency Care — Clothing, Financial, Food and Shelter. Agencies as well as churches and synagogues provide for emergency necessities. Contact the local Area Agency on Aging for available emergency facilities.

72-Hour Hold. In some states and localities a physician along with other professionals can place a temporary restraining order on a patient when he/she is considered dangerous to himself/herself or another person or is gravely disabled. The physician calls a hospital or psychiatric institution and informs them that he is placing a restraint on a patient. He then writes a prescription describing the patient's situation and the patient is transported to the hospital (usually against his will). After 72 hours, the attending physician will attempt to convince the patient to sign himself/herself into the hospital, if still appropriate. If the patient refuses, the physician can file a certification process in which a hearing is held to resolve the situation. The patient must remain in the hospital until the hearing is complete.

Medical

A patient may need medical services over and above those offered by a primary physician. Some services have branches dedicated to the concerns of older people. The following is a list of specialized medical services available, some of which offer special discounts for the elderly.

Services for the Blind. Twelve percent of older people are blind with an additional eight percent having chronic vision impairments. If a patient needs assistance with mobility and activities of daily living because of vision impairments, organizations are available to help older people function better in their surroundings. These services can provide talking books and seeing eye dogs, give instruction on special cooking techniques and much more. Contact the National Society to Prevent Blindness or the American Council of the Blind for details.

Dental Care. Proper dental care is important to proper nutrition. People cannot chew food such as meat and fresh vegetables without partials or dentures. Although dentures and partials can be costly, some clinics and offices offer discounts to seniors. Prices can vary considerably, so encourage older patients to shop around for the best price. Some areas may have vans that go out to the home-bound elderly to provide dental services. Call the Area Agency on Aging for more specific information or look in the Yellow Pages under "Dentists' Referral and Information Services."

Nutritional and Diabetic Counseling. Eating well-balanced meals contributes to physical as well as mental health. Nutritional specialists at local hospitals offer educational and motivational classes on well-balanced diets. Call a local hospital to find out what programs are available.

Hearing Care. Good hearing is an essential part of communication. Call the National Information Center on Deafness or the National Association for Hearing and Speech Action for information on devices and local agencies which can aid the hearing impaired. (See CHAPTER 2 under "Options for the Hearing Impaired" for more details.)

Home Health Care. Home health care is medical assistance brought to the home. Medicare will pay for certain home care services when provided under a physician's orders. Services provided under a home health care program include:
— Nursing Care
— Physical Therapy
— Occupational Therapy
— Speech and Hearing Therapy
— Medical Social Work
— Homemaker Services

Contact the National Association of Homecare or the American Federation of Home Health for local contacts.

Emergency Response Systems. The Emergency Response System was established for people who live alone or who are left alone most of the time. A small boxlike transmitting device is worn on the person. If the person has an emergency, such as a fall or a heart problem, he or she can activate the alarm by pushing a button. When activated, the system automatically calls a hospital or police station. The hospital or police designee then contacts the patient via telephone. If the person who activated the alarm does not answer the phone, an ambulance is sent to the home to assist. Call a local hospital or the Area Agency on Aging for more information.

Substance Abuse Treatment. Older alcoholics can often be categorized in two types—early or late onset. Early onset alcoholics have been drinking or abusing substances for years while late onset alcoholics have just begun to abuse substances. Alcohol and drug treatment centers often have divisions which focus special attention toward older people and their special substance abuse problems. Contact the National Clearing House for Alcohol and Drug Information or the local Alcoholics Anonymous chapter for further direction.

Supportive Devices/Equipment/Supplies. Many medical supply stores will comply with a physician's orders, bill Medicare and/or Medicaid if applicable, and deliver needed equipment to the patient's home the same day. Check with several local suppliers before ordering equipment.

CHAPTER 5
Geriatric Facility Design Considerations

Sensory perception (smell, touch, vision and hearing) and physical ability (level of frailness and response speed) decline with age. The decline can cause frustration and confusion in the elderly, especially in a society designed and built for a younger population.

Professionals in the field of aging should be aware of existing environmental structures and should note modifications which can be made to fit the needs of the elderly. These changes should improve functional ability for seniors and also improve the environmental accessibility for all age groups.

Most offices will not be able to adopt all of the recommendations presented in this chapter. However, some modifications, both minor and major, can be implemented during renovations to any physician's office or during the development of a new office.

Acoustics

Background noise and poor acoustics can contribute to listening difficulties, triggering increased frustration and agitation. To reduce noise in a hectic environment the following suggestions may be appropriate.

- Use sound absorbing surfaces and textured walls such as sheet rubber, heavy duty vinyl and carpeting.

- If possible, replace noisy machines, (i.e., mechanical ventilating/heating units, copy machine, centrifuge) with newer, less noisy ones or relocate them away from patient care areas.

- If noisy machines cannot be replaced or relocated, baffle adjacent walls with fire-rated panels or fire-rated soft wall types of material and/or area dividers.

- Separate conversational areas from noisy front desk area or nursing stations. Sturdy area dividers can be used, if walls are not present.

- Eliminate invisible, unpredictable sources of noise (e.g., piped in music, ceiling mounted public address systems).

- If a piped-in music system is used, tune to a station which features soothing instrumental music.

- To page staff or to transfer calls, use in-house telephone call systems rather than a public address system.

Illumination/Glare

Poor lighting and/or excessive glare can contribute to a loss of balance and increased falls. To control reflective glare, the following may be implemented.

- Use non-glare paint and matte wall coverings everywhere when repainting.

- Use light tones on walls to increase the impact of lighting fixtures.

- Cover windows with various window coatings (tinted glass, mylarlike shades, vertical blinds, etc.) to avoid glare.

- Replace or shade fixtures which have exposed bulbs.

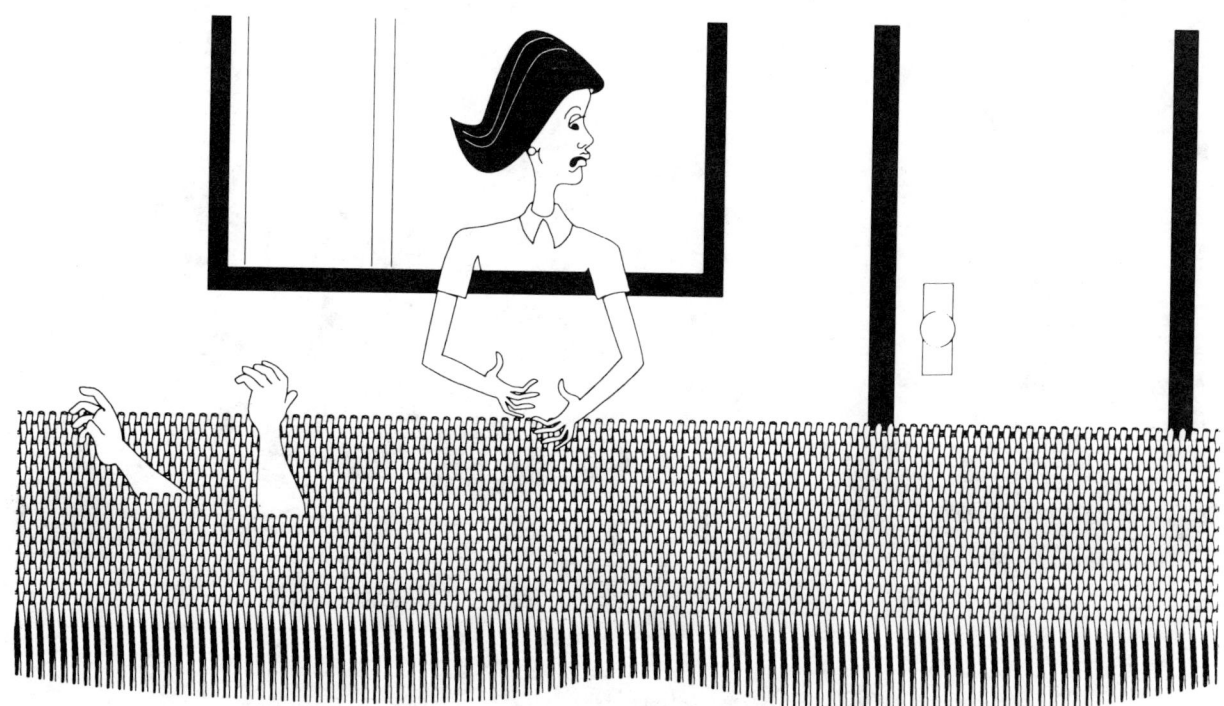

"Dr. Rovig, you're wonderfully plush new carpet seems to have swallowed your 10 o'clock appointment."

Use of Color/Pattern/Texture

Older people require about three times as much light to perceive colors with the same brilliance as seen during their younger years. A good way to test how a chosen color looks to many older people is to look through a piece of amber glass or yellow/brown acetate when judging wall tones and colored surfaces. Other hints are:

- Use light colors. However be aware that colors of similar intensity, brightness or dullness are more difficult for seniors to differentiate when used together under similar light conditions.

- Use ceiling level stripes or border prints, especially if your office has long hallways.

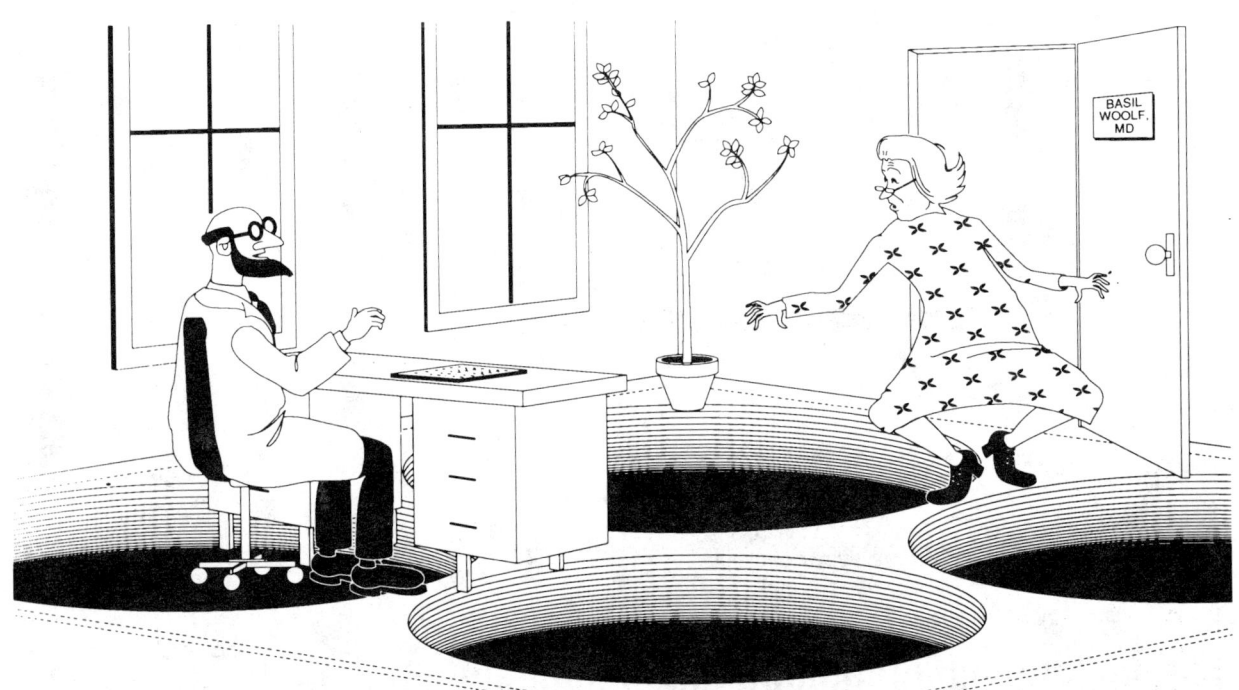

"So, Mrs. Bobbin, don't you just love the pattern on my new Swedish carpet?"

- Avoid wavy patterns or those that appear to be in motion. Bold diagonal stripes may look like stairways, causing confusion.

- White, although thought of as an 'institutional' color, is still a good contrasting color and is an especially good background color for wallhangings, artwork, etc.

Flooring

Older people are likely to have diminished depth perception. They may not perceive color patterns on the floor as a smooth level surface. Floor patterns can also camouflage such things as table legs, chair legs, canes, walkers and even feet, making tripping incidents more common. For both safety and aesthetics:

- Avoid uneven or slippery surfaces (e.g., ceramic tile in bathrooms).

- Avoid all unnecessary floor patterns, especially those that appear to vibrate.

- Avoid using throw rugs. They are dangerous and can cause tripping. Throw rugs should either be removed or firmly tacked down.

- Solid colors and non-skid surfaces are best.

Carpeting

Carpeting should be considered for its contribution to the overall feel of the environment. In addition, carpeting can improve the visual environment by reducing glare and lending to security and stability for walking. It also cushions the impact of sound waves contributing to better overall acoustics of the room and contributes to energy savings through greater heat retention. While minimizing the risk of falls, carpeting also causes less injury to patients if falls do occur. When selecting carpeting, be aware of the following.

- Select carpeting with antimicrobial finishes to protect against bacterial growth and eliminate odor and mildew.

- Look for finishes which provide protection against stains and static especially in waiting room areas and busy hallways.

- Improved nylons and herculon are good fibers to use; olefin is less expensive than nylon and resists mildew and will not absorb much moisture but does have a tendency to show tracking.

- Look for impermeable, nondegradable backings.

- Install carpeting with Class A, Type 1 fire rating only for public areas, both in face and backing materials.

- Height should be limited to 1/8" to 1/4"; face weight approximately 24 ounces.

- The surface should consist of level loops which allow for smooth transport of wheelchairs; avoid sculptures and shags.

- Use medium color tones which make stains and dirt less visible; contrast the wall color with the floor color (but not to an extreme); small patterns are acceptable, but watch out for those that vibrate.

- Pads are not advisable; glued carpeting is less likely to shift.

- For carpet on stairs, use ribbed vinyl or rubber stair nosing of a contrasting color for safety.

Grab Rails

Decreased mobility in seniors draws attention to the many hazards of everyday surroundings. Grab rails are an essential, low-cost precaution which can be taken to avoid some of the hazards. Good placement is as important as the grab rails.

- Grab rails should be mounted on two sides of the walls especially in toilet rooms, along all hallways and anywhere existing floors are hazardous.

- Rails should be well-balanced, horizontal grabbing surfaces.

- Surfaces should be solid like the armrest of a chair.

Furniture

Poorly designed, unbalanced and erratically placed furniture can be another source of disorientation and frustration for geriatric patients. Maneuverability and overall functioning can be deterred by the layout of a room, especially for those confined to wheelchairs. Elements to bear in mind for comprehensive room planning include:

- Height of furniture is important. The patients' feet need to be supported on the ground.

- Be cautious of overstuffed chairs and couches. Furniture should be comfortable, yet also be firm enough to give balance to the patient who has trouble maneuvering.

- Straight and wing-back chairs provide more support and allow for a variety of torso positions.

Chapter 5   Geriatric Facility Design Considerations   49

- Eliminate excessive furniture. Room layouts should take into account extra space needed for wheelchair patients.

- Eliminate low or sharp-edged coffee or end tables as they may cause additional hazards to those with limited sight or mobility. Round tables are best.

- A coffee pot, fruit and a water dispenser can make a patient's wait more comfortable.

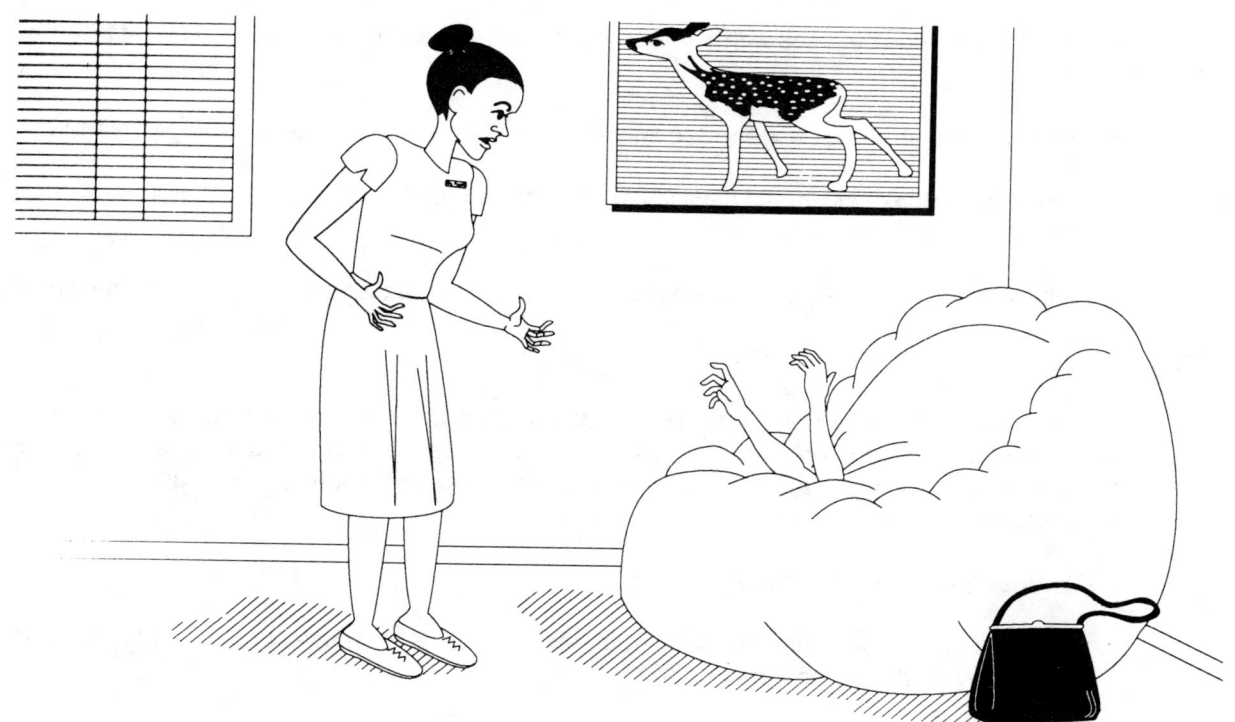

"Mrs. Longley, I'm supposed to warn you not to sit in the overstuffed chair. Mrs. Longley?"

Entryway/Lobby

Entrances portray the atmosphere of a physician's practice. Easy access and pleasant settings can instill a positive mood and help contribute to a more comfortable visit for the patient. Suggested improvements for the entryway or lobby are:

- Provide sloping ramps and sliding, automatic glass doors where possible. If this isn't possible, at least make sure the door is lightweight and is fairly easy to open.

- Provide handrails next to the entryways if floor surface is slippery.

- Make sure entry paths and sidewalks are wide enough to accommodate wheelchairs.

- Provide curbside benches with armrests near steps so people can go up or down at their own pace.

- Plants along entry paths, near doorways or in waiting areas convey a feeling of warmth.

- The information desk should have lower areas for wheelchair access; good acoustics in this area are important.

- Outside steps and entryways can be painted with gritty weather-proof paint to prevent falling.

Art

Art can play several roles in a physician's office. It can be used as a point of comfort, anchoring older people to the present. Familiar art can be used as a means of judging alertness and stimulating easier conversation. Several points to be aware of when selecting art for an office include:

- Images should be identifiable.

- Textured pieces, 3-dimensional (e.g., mobiles at windows) or textiles placed strategically are especially useful as focal points.

- Groupings of pictures add a comfortable feeling to a room.

- Borrowed exhibits from local artists, seniors groups or local museums add the dimension of change to the facility, stimulating conversation and catering to the various tastes of the patients. They can also be an easy way to redecorate without added strain on the budget.

Signage

Because colors are abstract, they should be used minimally when signifying different areas within a setting. Signs, objects and textures are better used for orientation purposes than colors. However, a blend of colors, objects and signage can be useful.

- Colors may be used to signify change, suggest edging or they may emphasize contours. Themes can be repeated throughout the facility to signal specific areas such as exam rooms and bathrooms.

- Colors can also be used to camouflage areas, e.g., exam room or nurse stations. Doorways may be painted the same color as the walls.

- Signage must be within the visual range of an older person. By using symbols rather than words, the elderly are better able to distinguish meanings. Also, symbols can be seen at greater distances.

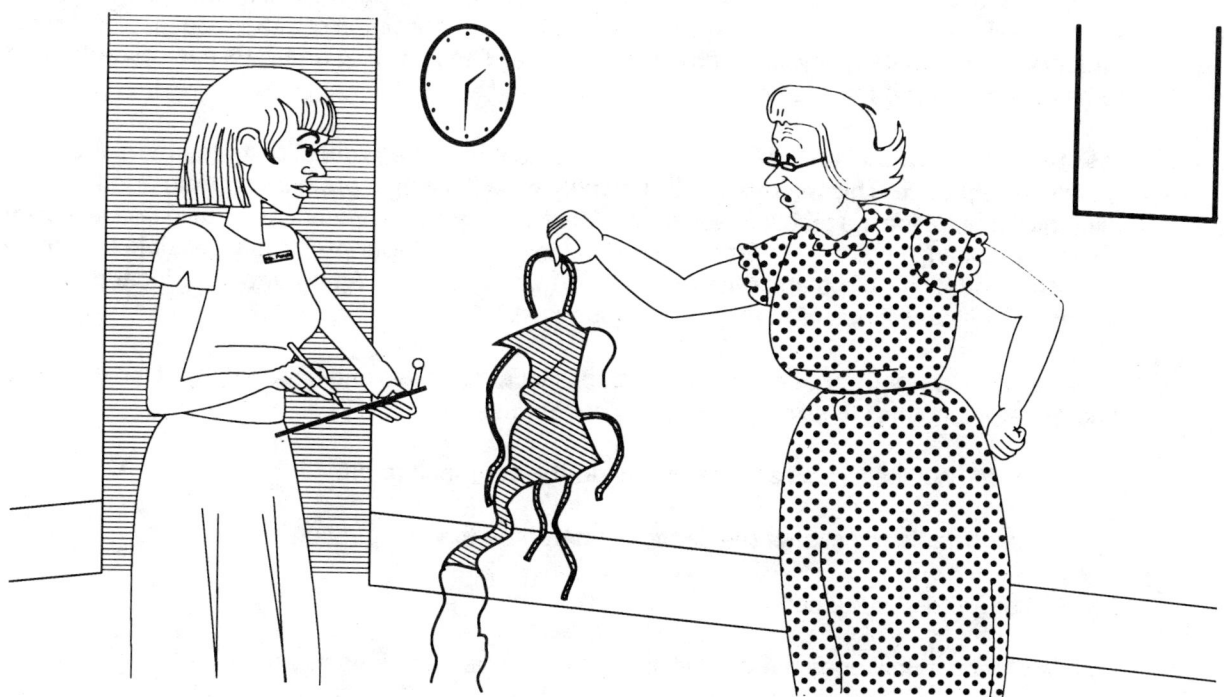

"You said you were going to give me an examination gown and then you handed me this kite instead."

CHAPTER 6
Marketing to the Geriatric Population

A marketing strategy involves everything from a friendly smile to a sophisticated advertising campaign. Each new service added to a practice should serve to advertise and market the practice. The most effective promotion is word of mouth from a satisfied patient. There are many different methods of marketing a practice ranging from simple tips that can be implemented with a small marketing budget, to a large advertising campaign focused on achieving the broadest possible exposure. The strategy contained in this marketing section is generic and meant to be adaptable to different communities.

Demographics

A basic understanding of the market is essential prior to development of any marketing strategy. Demographic information should be collected to identify the location of current patients, potential patients and competing physician practice locations. The following analyses can be performed to better understand the market served.

Identify the Potential Market. Compare the medical practice population to the market by age group and zip code. This information will identify where patients are coming from and the level of market penetration the practice represents. Targeted marketing approaches can increase market share. By locating senior high-rises, community centers and apartments it is possible to identify high concentrations of potential patients. The Area Agency on Aging and your local planning department have listings of these concentrations.

Analyze the Competition. Competition includes local hospitals and/or other physician practices and geriatric centers. To size up your competition, use the four P's listed below.

Product: What services and programs do the competition provide?

Price: What is the cost of the services offered by the competition?

Place: Where is the competition located?

Promotion: How does the competition promote their services or programs?

Strategies. While there are numerous possible marketing strategies, four are particularly relevant to discuss in connection with promoting physician practices.

Innovation: Take risks, set up new services presently not available in the market.

Joint Venture: Locate other providers desiring to enter new service areas and together share the cost of initiating this new service or program. A joint venture may be with another physician's office or a local hospital.

Status Quo: Do not add any new services.

Elimination: If the competition can do it cheaper and better, let them.

Media

Many types of media can be utilized to increase and maintain awareness in the community. The effectiveness of the promotional material chosen can be measured by asking new patients how they were referred to the practice. A special phone line with a unique phone number could be utilized to isolate the calls generated from a radio commercial or a particular printed piece.

Print. Print advertising is relatively inexpensive and provides high visibility to a targeted group. Various types of print material could be appropriate for each practice. Brochures and pamphlets include general information and are usually kept by individuals for reference purposes. Flyers are used to announce special events and should be concise, short and hard hitting. Newsletters, produced on a regular basis, can contain health education information and can also introduce new staff and new services.

When developing printed material specifically for the older population, certain techniques should be considered to promote the highest level of interest.

- *Color contrast* between the ink color and the paper color is very important. Black ink on contrasting paper such as white, ivory or yellow is recommended. Blue, green and violet colors should be avoided. Several studies suggest that the lens of the eye yellows with age and filters out the blue end of the light spectrum. Colors which are easier for older adults to distinguish include yellows, oranges and reds.

- *Large print size* such as 14 point is recommended for material that is written for older adults. Newspapers in most cities use 10 point print targeted for the general population with 20/20 eyesight. As the eye ages, the lens diminishes in its ability to see close objects. More than half of the over-65 population have the visual acuity of 20/70. Older adults will not read material if it strains their eyes. Therefore, the use of 14 point print will encourage older adults to read your material.

- *Simple type faces* such as Universe, Goudy Bold or Times-Roman increase legibility. Fancy typefaces may have the opposite effect. A printer can provide examples of the numerous typefaces available for publications.

- *Dull paper* or semi-gloss paper should be used whenever possible. High gloss paper produces glare and can be difficult for seniors to read.

- Use *simple clear language* and avoid medical terminology such as osteoporosis, oncology, cardiology and ophthalmology. The terms "arthritis," "cancer," "heart" and "eye care" better communicate with your audience.

- *Photographs* add warmth to a brochure or pamphlet. Photos of the clinic, the staff and patients can enhance the appearance of the brochure.

- The more *colorful* your material is the more attractive it may be. However, use of multiple colors can greatly increase cost.

- *Ink sketches* or *cartoons* can also be effective. They are less expensive to print than photographs and are often the first point of contact between the material and the reader's eye.

- Too much information can clutter your material. Leave a large amount of *open space* throughout the piece.

- The *name* and the *phone number* of the clinic should be highly visible. A *map* with major landmarks designated can make a practice easier to find.

Printers base their price on the number of total pieces printed. Printing in larger quantities reduces the cost per piece. Most of the print cost is in typesetting and press setup.

Direct Mail. Many corporations and businesses use direct mail to attract new customers or to notify customers of new services or special programs. Direct mail should elicit response from potential customers. A targeted approach to these interested parties can often make a sale.

By providing a prepaid response card, potential customers can request specific information. The easier it is for the potential customer, the more likely the response. A two percent return rate is considered a good response to direct mailings. Some points to keep in mind when preparing a direct mailing are:

- Ask the local postmaster how to set up prepaid return postage for the direct mail piece.

- To avoid the necessity of an envelope, use 80 to 100 pound stock paper.

- For small mailings, stamps can be used. Larger mailings may necessitate the purchase of a bulk mail permit from the post office. The permit number is then preprinted on the direct mail piece.

- Postage costs are reduced if direct bulk mail is presorted by zip code, marked by stickers and placed in mailbags.

- If a computerized database of patients is not used within the practice, a commercial mailing service can develop a database and generate mailing labels in zip code order. The mailing service could also be employed to sort labels generated by the practice in other than zip code order.

Articles. Articles published in local journals, magazines and newspapers give the practice increased recognition in the community. They also may increase the practice's referral base from professionals in the community as well as enlighten older adults who read the articles.

Radio. Radio is a good marketing medium to use to reach a specifically targeted age group such as seniors. Arbitron ratings can identify the top three stations listened to by people 65 and over. (See Exhibit 8 on page 60 for a sample Arbitron rating sheet.) A media buyer or radio station should be contacted to obtain the ratings results. The cost of the air time depends on the time of day the advertisement is aired. The cost per airing is reduced as the number of spots aired is increased. For maximum market penetration, a minimum airing of three times per week for six weeks is recommended. It is unnecessary to change the spot during this period.

Radio commercials can be written by anyone familiar with the practice, or an agency can be hired to develop the script. Radio station personnel can also assist with the script. A 30-second spot is usually appropriate unless the subject matter requires more explanation.

The radio spot can be taped at the radio station for no additional cost if time is bought. Usually the station manager allows the person producing the spot to announce it. A professional at the radio station is always available to announce the spot if the advertiser does not have an available person to speak. If possible, try to tape your own spot. A new voice on the air will attract the audience's attention.

Public Service Announcements. Public Service Announcements (PSAs) are available for free to nonprofit organizations and for community events sponsored by nonprofit organizations. All radio stations must air PSAs as part of their licensing agreement. However, because of the volume of announcements sent to radio stations, there is no guarantee that a particular PSA will be aired, and, if it is aired, it may be given a time slot in the middle of the night. A script should be sent to the radio station and the spot will be read by the announcer. Following are examples of 30-second public service announcements.

Don't leave your pharmacy without the most important ingredient: knowledge. Your pharmacist is trained to answer your questions about your medications. By becoming more informed about your prescription medications you will be able to avoid side effects and get the most out of the medications you take. This message is a community service of Dr. _____'s office.

Studies show that about half of all prescription drugs are taken incorrectly. Half! Your medicines cannot help you unless you take them correctly. Be sure to follow the directions for use exactly. This message is a community service of Dr. _____ _____ office.

Talk Shows. Schedule guest appearances on radio talk shows. Radio stations are always eager to identify new ideas and new subject matters. Use a local hospital's public relations department to contact a radio station for scheduling appearances. If the community does not have a radio show geared toward health issues or the needs of older adults, consider starting one.

Television. Television is the most expensive form of advertising and is a "shot gun" approach, reaching the general market, but not a specifically targeted group. Older adults watch more daytime television than younger adults. Placing ads during the daytime time slots between 10:00 am and 6:00 pm will reach the greatest number of seniors. Advertising is also less expensive during these time slots. The news hour is more expensive, but is also a good time to reach older adults.

If an experienced producer is not available within the practice, the television studio or a production company can produce the spot for an additional fee. The cost per spot will vary by the time of the spot and the number of viewers watching the station. The more times a spot airs, the greater the market reach. Cost also decreases proportionately to the number of spots aired. Independent stations are less expensive than the national networks. Cost should be considered on the basis of price per 1000 viewers.

Nielsen ratings will determine the channel and program which most effectively target the senior market. Each television station can provide the Nielsen ratings for their programs. Other marketing research may also be available from the television stations.

Public Service Announcements. Nonprofit organizations and community events sponsored by nonprofit organizations get free recognition from television. Usually a script or ideas are sent to the television station of choice along with slides and a video, if available. The television station may or may not air the PSA, depending on available air time. PSAs are often aired in the wee morning hours. There is no cost to the organization for air time.

Local Talk Shows and News Programs. Send information regarding the practices' senior services to local talk shows that include topics of interest to seniors in their programming. Ask to be placed on their speakers' list. When a program coincides with the practices' expertise, the station will most likely call. Whenever new services are initiated, let the television talk shows and news programs know. If it is a hot topic, the practice may receive news coverage.

Other Community Advertising. Community advertising provides a permanent identification of the practice's location in the community. This form of advertising is relatively inexpensive and allows high visibility if appropriately placed.

- *Clinic Signs.* A large sign should always be placed outside the door which can be easily read. If the clinic is located within the hospital or medical building, multiple signs may be necessary.

- *Bus Benches.* Bus bench advertising should be placed in front of large senior high-rises or senior centers located near the physician's practice on a major street.

- *Billboard Signs.* Advertisements can be placed on billboards close to the practice or near high density senior neighborhoods.

- *Bus Advertising.* Signs identifying the practice are particularly effective on buses which travel routes close to the practice.

- *Clinic Vehicle.* A handicap-equipped van and a van driver are wonderful marketing tools for the practice as well as a means to bring patients to and from the clinic. Advertise by painting the name of the practice on the side of the vehicle.

- *Supermarket Signs.* More and more supermarkets are providing stands for community advertisements. A sign should be placed at supermarkets which cater to a large senior population.

The Little Extras

In addition to the more conventional (and expensive) marketing approaches presented above, seniors are particularly receptive to the little extras described below.

Health Fairs. A health fair is a forum for free preventive health screenings and tests which are made available to the public as a community service and to promote good health. A health fair can be sponsored by the practice or in conjunction with a local hospital or other practices or local businesses including television and radio stations. It involves a lot of work, so the more participants the easier it will be.

Health fairs should provide preventive health screenings free of charge to the participants. A minimum fee could be charged for some specialized tests. The following services may be offered at a health fair:
- Eye tests - screenings for glaucoma
- Blood pressure tests
- Anemia tests
- Hearing tests
- Colon screenings
- Glucose tests
- Cholesterol tests
- Foot care

Contact the Area Agency on Aging or the United Way for listings of agencies that may wish to be included in a health fair. Numerous social service agencies may wish to contribute.
- Meals on Wheels
- American Heart Association
- American Stroke Association
- Social Security Administration - Medicare

To staff the health fair, the entire practice can participate for the day, or temporary labor can be hired to administer the screenings. Using the physicians may enhance the overall success of the health fair. As participants become familiar with a physician they will often schedule appointments with that individual.

The health fair may be located at a variety of sites:

- The *physicians' office* may be used if space permits. The physicians may consider closing for the day or for half a day to accommodate the health fair.

- A *senior center* where seniors normally congregate for the noon meal may be used. A listing of senior centers can be found in the governmental section of the phone book under "Parks and Recreation Facilities" or under "Senior Services."

- *Shopping malls* may be used for larger health fairs. Many managers are eager to sponsor a health fair which will attract new people to the mall for the day.

- *Banks* may also be used. Many banks have started senior clubs and are interested in attracting new senior members to their bank. The health fair can be scheduled on the third day of the month which is when seniors usually deposit their social security checks.

To publicize the health fair, newspaper ads, articles, direct mail and flyers may be used. Banks and shopping malls will also assist in marketing the event.

Community Presentations. Seniors can be invited to the office to attend free health education programs, or health education programs can be offered free of charge at senior high-rises, senior centers and churches. Presentations can also be made to senior organizations such as the American Association of Retired Persons or the Retired Teachers Association. Refreshments can be served and brochures, flyers and giveaways (i.e., key chains, jar openers) should be handed out at the end of the program. Advertise in local newspapers and the clinic newsletter. If the program is offered outside of the clinic, the facility should promote the program through their own newsletters and bulletins. Suggested community contacts and possible sites include:
- Home health care agencies
- Public health programs
- Church leaders and other leaders in the community

- American Association of Retired Persons
- Directors of senior centers
- Managers of senior high-rises
- Retired Teachers Association
- Veterans' Administration
- Alzheimer's Disease and Related Disorders Association
- American Cancer Society
- Diabetes Association
- Political groups such as senior lobbies
- Politicians; local, state and federal
- Insurance carriers
- Geriatrics Society

Cards. Birthday cards can be sent out to each patient every year. A card will mean a great deal to the elderly patient who may live alone and to those without family or social supports. The birthday card from the clinic may be the only birthday acknowledgement the patient receives. Also, sympathy cards can be sent to the family of a patient who dies.

Special Patient Gifts. Patients enjoy receiving small free gifts from their physician. Patients will tell their friends about the uniqueness of the practice. The gift can be printed with the clinic's name, address and phone number to publicize the practice. Some gift ideas are:
- Refrigerator magnets
- Jar openers
- Holiday cookies
- Magnifying glasses

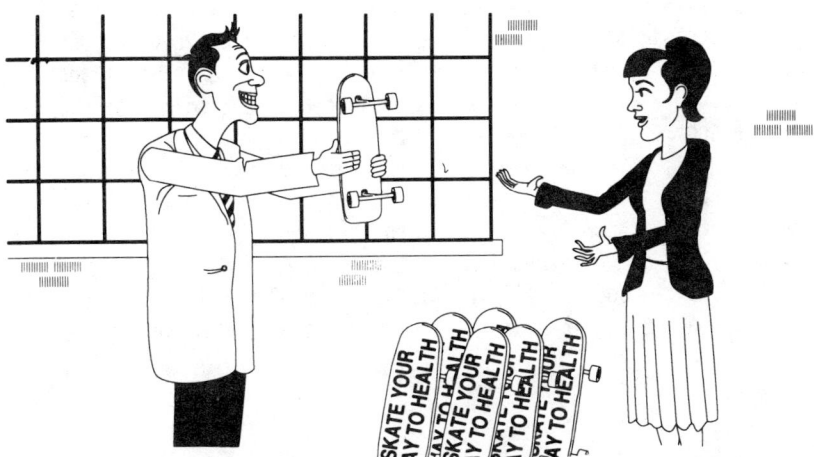

"It's certainly a novel approach, Dr. Mobstock, but do you really think your geriatric patients would respond to free promotional skateboards?"

Exhibit 8
Arbitron Ratings

Strata Super Ranker
Top 10 Stations: Cume and AQH Ranked on Cume
Demographic: Adults 50+

Market: Denver-Boulder Metro
Population: 376,400
Arbitron Fall 1988

Rk	Saturday 3pm-7pm			Rk	Saturday 7pm-mid			Rk	Sunday 6am-10am		
	Station	Cume	AQH		Station	Cume	AQH		Station	Cume	AQH
1	OSI/EZW	49,400	18,400	1	KOA -AM	26,600	9,400	1	OSI/EZW	45,300	17,300
2	KYGO-FM	14,700	5,800	2	OSI/EZW	22,600	6,200	2	KOA -AM	28,300	8,700
3	KOA -AM	14,000	4,500	3	KYGO-FM	8,000	1,800	3	KYGO-AF	21,600	12,400
4	KVOD-FM	8,500	2,700	4	KVOD-FM	5,200	1,300	4	KYGO-FM	14,700	7,800
5	KYGO-AM	5,200	2,700	5	KDEN-AM	4,800	800	5	KDEN-AM	12,800	2,600
6	KHOW-AM	4,800	1,500	6	KZRZ-FM	4,300	1,000	6	KHOW-AM	10,300	4,500
7	KDEN-AM	4,000	1,000	7	KLZ -AM	4,000	1,300	7	KVOD-FM	9,400	3,600
8	KRKS-AM	3,100	700	8	KHOW-AM	2,200	800	8	KLZ -AM	7,300	2,600
9	KRXY-AF	3,000	2,500	9	KRXY-AF	1,600	200	9	KYGO-AM	7,100	4,600
10	KRXY-FM	3,000	2,500	10	KRXY-FM	1,600	200	10	KDKO-AM	5,000	2,400

CHAPTER 7
Geriatric Legal and Ethical Issues

Discussing legal and ethical areas of concern with patients can be a very difficult yet important task for the physician. Three topics most often discussed are the living will, guardianship and the revocation of an elderly patient's driver's license.

Living Will

A living will is a document that allows a person to state in advance decisions regarding his or her health care. In the event of a terminal illness or irreversible condition, the living will document directs the physician whether or not to use heroic measures to keep the patient alive if the patient's death is imminent. The meaning of the term "heroic measures" varies depending on the laws in each particular state. For example, it may or may not include the withdrawal of food or hydration, depending on the statute. Living wills (also called advance directives) are designed to:

- Allow a competent adult to make health care decisions in advance of incapacity. Some states provide for designation of a proxy within the declaration itself.

- Give physicians the opportunity to implement their patients' health care wishes under statutory authority without the threat of criminal or civil liability.

As of June 1989, all but 10 states have enacted "living will" statutes. The states which have no laws concerning living wills include (* indicates pending legislation):

Kentucky	*New York
*Massachusetts	*Ohio
*Michigan	*Pennsylvania
*Nebraska	Rhode Island
*New Jersey	South Dakota

Many states have enacted a "Durable Power of Attorney" for Health Care. This document allows a competent person to appoint another person to make medical decisions for him or her in the event of future incapacity.

What can a physician do to aid his patient with the process?

- Call or write the Society for the Right to Die at 250 West 57th Street, New York, NY 10107, (212) 246-6973 for a copy of the living will form in statute language appropriate for the state of residence. Also, request the guidelines for its proper execution. In those states that still lack legislation, the Society provides "Living Will Declaration" forms in general language.

- Have living will forms available for patients in the office. (See Exhibit 9 on page 66 for an example.)

- Become familiar with the form so an explanation can be given to patients if they are interested in a living will.

- Suggest to all patients that they make their health care wishes known to their physicians, family and friends.

- Encourage patients to provide an original living will form for their medical charts, discuss this with family members or friends and give them a copy and keep one with their important documents.

- To facilitate the identification of patients who have signed living wills, stamp the words "LIVING WILL" on the outside of the chart.

- Most important—physicians should be aware of their patients' wishes in the event of a catastrophic illness.

The subject of living wills can be an uncomfortable subject to discuss for both the physician and the patient. Some patients may want to discuss the issue in-depth, while others may not want to talk about it at all. Listen for the patient's reaction and respond accordingly.

A good way to approach the subject may be to ask the patient if they know about living wills and what they do. Also, explain to the patient that as his physician, you want to be clear about the feelings he or she may have in regard to living wills. Often, the patient will be more apt to discuss living wills or the issues of death and dying than the medical professional. Make the patient understand there is no right answer. The decision to have a living will is a decision only the patient can make.

Guardianship

Guardianships are designed to protect and provide care to those who are unable to manage their own affairs. Guardianships, sometimes called conservatorships, are available in all states. A guardianship/conservatorship is a legal ruling that gives another person (family member, friend, state worker or other) control over the financial and personal affairs of an incapacitated person. The Uniform Probate Code defines an incapacitated person as, "One who is impaired by reason of mental illness, mental deficiency, illness or disability, advanced age, chronic use of drugs, chronic intoxication or other cause (except minority) to the extent lacking sufficient understanding or capacity to make or communicate responsible decisions."

Since guardianship is expensive, cumbersome and results in a drastic loss of basic rights for the ward, it should be used only as a last resort. Physicians can play an important role in preventing the need for guardianship by encouraging their patients to execute a health care power of attorney. This document enables a patient to appoint another person to make any or all health care decisions, and to spell out guidelines for those decisions if the patient becomes incapacitated.

However, many patients fail to make such arrangements in advance. Thus, physicians may become involved in the guardianship process. Their involvement may be in two ways. First, the physician may question the patient's capacity to give informed consent for medical treatment, and may initiate consideration of guardianship. If the physician feels the patient needs a guardian to make health care decisions, he or she should:

- Try to talk to the patient about guardianship and what it does. Ask the patient who he or she feels would be an appropriate guardian (i.e., a person the patient trusts and with whom he or she feels comfortable).

- Call the family member or friend the patient referred to and discuss the need for a guardianship.

- If the patient is not able to understand the guardianship concept, call a member of his or her family and discuss the need for a guardianship.

- If the patient has no relative or friend who is willing to be appointed as a guardian, call the county social service adult unit and discuss the case with a staff member on the unit. Some localities have public or private guardianship agencies.

Second, the physician may be asked to provide a written statement to the court—and sometimes to testify—regarding a patient's medical condition. Some courts have forms for the physician's statement. (See Exhibit 10 on pages 67 and 68.) In order to provide the judge with the most thorough and accurate information, it will be important to describe concisely:
— Patient's medical history, and length of physician's professional relationship with patient
— Date patient was last seen, length of time and tests performed
— Effects of nutrition, medication, emotional state, metabolic factors, etc., on patient's condition
— Diagnosis and prognosis, and whether condition is fluctuating or constant
— Comments on how patient's condition may affect those functional abilities in question (to make and communicate decisions, to maintain personal hygiene, to maintain proper diet, maintain personal safety, etc.)

Do not make a conclusory statement about the patient's legal capacity or about the need for a guardianship. That is the job of the judge. Remember that guardianship takes rights away from people. Although often necessary, a guardianship appointment can be a devastating loss of independence to the patient.

Revocation of Driver's License

A driver's license is a ticket to independence for both old and young. Without a license, a person feels less in control of his life.

Older people may be at risk of losing their licenses due to seizures, strokes, failing eyesight or hearing or even for having slower reaction time. The authority to revoke a driver's license lies with the Department of Motor Vehicles. They usually act on the recommendation of the Department of Transportation's Medical Advisory Board if a medical condition is the cause. The Medical Advisory Board receives requests for possible revocation from three places: 1) a physician can refer a patient; 2) a family member can refer another family member (the request must be notarized); or 3) if the driver's license renewal staff detects a mental or physical disability, they can also refer to the medical board.

If a physician feels a patient is placing himself or other drivers in danger, he or she may choose to:

- Talk to the patient about the concerns regarding his or her driving.
- Talk to the family if possible.

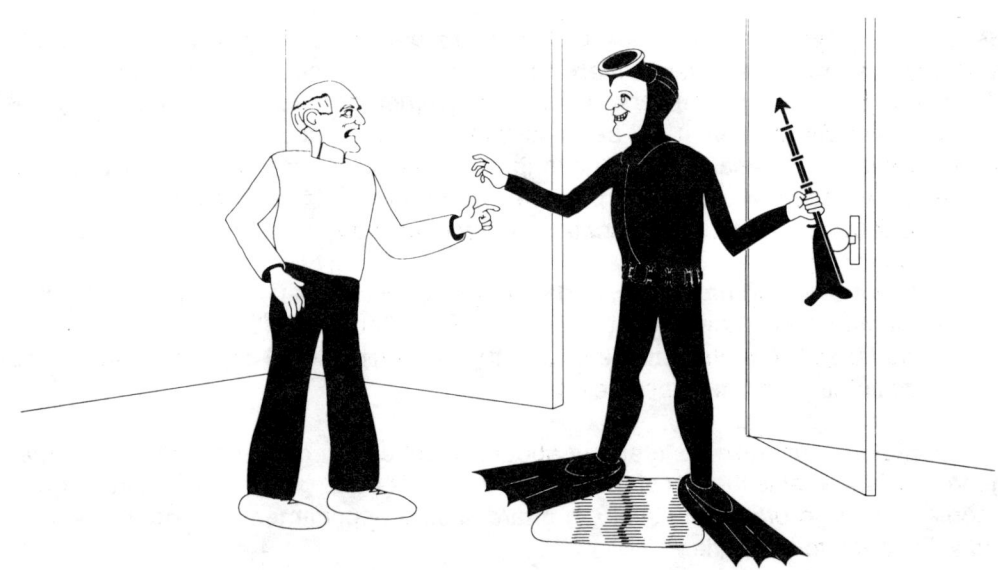

"I called the senior center because I need help DRIVING, knucklehead!"

Chapter 7   Geriatric Legal and Ethical Issues

- Tell the patient there may be alternatives to losing a license.

- Contact ADED, Association of Driver Educators for the Disabled, 33736 LaCross, Westland, Michigan 48185, (313) 425-8911, for a list of evaluation centers in the area. This organization addresses driving issues for all special populations. ADED is an international organization which tries to discover what the person's deficit may be (i.e., slower reaction time) and tries to help the person compensate for it (i.e., adding another mirror, taking alternate routes or taking a driver's education class). There are many other suggestions and adaptive devices through this program. There is usually a fee for the service, which offers an unbiased view of the situation by a trained driver rehabilitation specialist.

- Call the Office of Driver Control at the Driver's License Bureau. This office is more likely to be less aware of alternatives to help a person compensate for his or her losses but may be a viable alternative. The Office of Driver Control will ask the physician to write a letter stating reasons for revocation.

    Taking a person's license can be a devastating experience. However, it is also important to make the roads safe for other drivers. Give the patient the benefit of the doubt and suggest they be retested before hastily suggesting revocation. Make sure to properly document the need for revocation in the medical record.

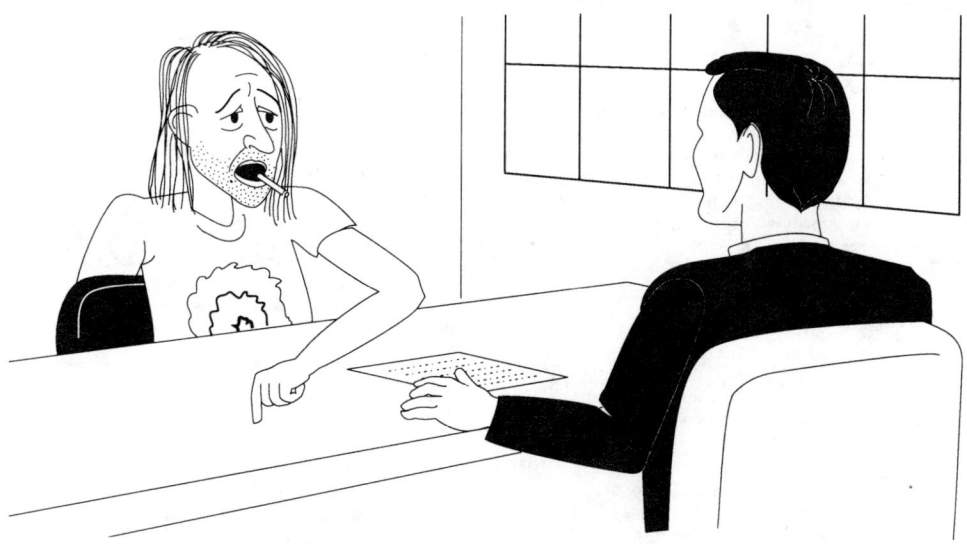

"Hello, I'm Harriet Goodson's living will, and I say she left everything to me."

Exhibit 9
Living Will

[SAMPLE]*

"LIVING WILL"

DECLARATION

Declaration made this _____ day of _____ 198___.

I, _____, being of sound mind, willfully and voluntarily make known my desires that my dying shall not be artificially prolonged under the circumstances set forth below, and do declare:

If at any time I should have an incurable injury, disease, or illness certified to be a terminal condition by two (2) physicians who have personally examined me, one of whom shall be my attending physician, and the physicians have determined that my death will occur whether or not life-sustaining procedures are utilized and where the application of life-sustaining procedures would serve only to artificially prolong the dying process, I direct that such procedures be withheld or withdrawn, and that I be permitted to die naturally with only the administration of medication or the performance of any medical procedure deemed necessary to provide me with comfort, care or to alleviate pain.

In the absence of my ability to give directions regarding the use of such life-sustaining procedures, it is my intention that this declaration shall be honored by my family and physician(s) as the final expression of my legal right to refuse medical or surgical treatment and accept the consequences from such refusal.

I understand the full import of this declaration and I am emotionally and mentally competent to make this declaration.

Signed _____
Address _____
_____

I believe the declarant to be of sound mind. I did not sign the declarant's signature above for or at the direction of the declarant. I am at least 18-years of age and am not related to the declarant by blood or marriage, entitled to any portion of the estate of the declarant according to the laws of intestate succession of the _____ or under any will of the declarant or codicil thereto, or directly financially responsible for declarant's medical care. I am not the declarant's attending physician, an employee of the attending physician, or an employee of the health facility in which the declarant is a patient.

Witness _____
Address _____
_____

Witness _____
Address _____
_____

ss.:

Before me, the undersigned authority, on this _____ day of _____, 198___, personally appeared _____, _____, and _____, known to me to be the Declarant and the witnesses, respectively, whose names are signed to the foregoing instrument, and who, in the presence of each other, did subscribe their names to the attached Declaration (Living Will) on this date, and that said Declarant at the time of execution of said Declaration was over the age of eighteen (18) years and of sound mind.

[SEAL]
My commission expires:

_____
Notary Public

*Check requirements of individual state statute.

Source: President's Commission for the Study of Ethical Problems in Medicine and Biobehavioral Research, "Deciding To Forego Life Sustaining Treatment," U.S. Government Printing Office, pages 314-315.

Exhibit 10
Physician's Evaluation/Conservatorship

PHYSICIAN'S EVALUATION/
CONSERVATORSHIP
PC-370 REV. 1/85
(PRC-84)

STATE OF CONNECTICUT
COURT OF PROBATE
[Type or Print]

Do not record

Court of Probate, District of	District No.

The undersigned physician states that he has personally examined said respondent and hereby makes his report as follows:

PHYSICIAN *[Name, address, zip code, and tel. no.]*	PRACTICING PSYCHIATRIST ☐ yes ☐ no
	CONN. MEDICAL LICENSE NO.
RESPONDENT *[Name]*	DATE OF EXAMINATION *[Mo., day, year]* *[Must be within 30 days preceding the hearing]*

Is the respondent suffering from a mental, emotional, or physical illness? ☐ yes ☐ no
If 'yes' answer all the following questions. You must give reasons for your opinions.

What specific type of mental, emotional or physical illness is involved?
Give diagnosis.

Does the respondent's mental, emotional, or physical condition have substantial adverse effects on his ability to function? Does the impairment affect the ability of the respondent in managing his affairs and/or his capability in caring for himself?

PERTINENT HISTORY

PHYSICAL CONDITION *[Describe physical impairments unless described in diagnosis above]*

PHYSICIAN'S EVALUATION/CONSERVATORSHIP

Exhibit 10 (continued)
Physician's Evaluation/Conservatorship

MENTAL CONDITION [Describe mental impairments unless described in diagnosis above].

ADDITIONAL COMMENTS:

I hereby certify that:

I am a licensed physician.
I have personally examined such Respondent on the aforementioned date.

DATE [Month, day, year]	SIGNED [Examining physician]

Note to physician: The following is the statutory requirement for the examination of the respondent.

At any hearing for involuntary representation, the court shall receive evidence regarding the condition of the respondent, including a written report or testimony by one or more physicians licensed to practice medicine in the state who have examined the respondent within thirty days preceding the hearing. The report or testimony shall contain specific information regarding the disability and the extent of its incapacitating effect.... If the court finds by clear and convincing evidence that the respondent is incapable of managing his or her affairs then the court shall appoint a conservator of such person's estate. If the court finds by clear and convincing evidence that the respondent is incapable of caring for himself or herself, then the court shall appoint a conservator of the person of the respondent.

CHAPTER 8
Successful Geriatric Programs

The Center for Research in Ambulatory Health Care Administration (CRAHCA), the research arm of Medical Group Management Association (MGMA), received a three-year grant in 1987 to demonstrate gerontology/geriatric programming in primary health care settings. The $1,199,889 million grant was funded by the W. K. Kellogg Foundation, Battle Creek, Michigan. Four demonstration sites were chosen for this project: Park Nicollet Medical Center of Minneapolis, Minnesota; The Duluth Clinic, Limited, of Duluth, Minnesota; The Honolulu Medical Group, Incorporated, in Honolulu, Hawaii; and Carle Clinic Association in Urbana, Illinois.

The four demonstration sites have changed their practices to be more sensitive to the needs of their elderly patients. Some of their successful programs are outlined below.

A packet of information including brochures and fliers on the programs developed at the four demonstration sites is available from CRAHCA for a nominal fee with the purchase of this book.

Park Nicollet Medical Center

Park Nicollet Medical Center (PNMC) is the fifth largest multispecialty group practice in the nation. Park Nicollet is composed of 256 physicians and 1,243 employees at 17 clinic sites in the Twin Cities area. Physicians at the Center represent 36 different specialties and subspecialties and see approximately 1.5 million patients every year. The Center is owned and governed by the physicians and is organized as a for-profit Minnesota corporation.

The Park Nicollet Medical Center has a strong commitment to gerontology. This interest is spurred by Park Nicollet's HMO Medicare risk contract to provide comprehensive medical care to approximately 7,000 seniors and supplemental care to an additional 2,000 seniors. Also, PNMC has approximately 315,000 straight Medicare visits annually, and provides nursing home primary care to over 1,200 institutionalized elderly.

Park Nicollet has implemented a number of successful programs which have enhanced the patient care rendered to their elderly clientele. Each program has a unique approach that has been successful in Minnesota and may be replicated in other communities.

Friendly Caller Program. The Friendly Caller Program provides socialization for frail elderly patients by utilizing volunteers to make social calls to patients. It has been successful in reducing the number of seniors who call in for non-medical reasons. Three volunteers call over 70 patients each week. The volunteers are supervised by the case manager. The case manager of the clinic

and a nurse also help supervise the volunteers. The supervisor provides the volunteer with some basic information about the patient, including:
- Name
- Marital status
- Age
- Number of children and grandchildren
- Hobbies or interests

The volunteers call the patient from the Medical Center and inform the patient they are calling on behalf of the Park Nicollet Medical Center. To protect confidentiality, the volunteers do not have access to the medical records. Volunteers meet with a supervisor weekly after the calls are made. If the volunteer notices a change in the patient, he or she notifies the supervisor who then may personally follow-up with the patient.

The friendly caller program has been a great success. Case managers report that the patients, many of whom live alone and are housebound are delighted to have social telephone chats. Families have also expressed appreciation. The volunteers have found the program rewarding and beneficial and are eager to see it continue to grow.

Over 50 and Fit Program. A peer-led low impact aerobic class called the "Over 50 and Fit Program" is offered at a local senior high-rise. The objectives of the exercise program are to maintain wellness attitudes, to perpetuate physical flexibility, stamina, and endurance and to promote inclinations toward self-care among the older population. A staff member at the Park Nicollet Medical Center taught a senior to lead the group through exercise routines with the assistance of instructors and a visual aid booklet.

Once the program was successfully operational, Park Nicollet Medical Center transferred the program from the Senior Services Department to the Health Education Department. The educational department has more resources to promote the Over 50 and Fit Program's growth.

Nursing Home Program. Park Nicollet serves approximately 1,000 nursing home patients in 67 homes throughout the metro area. Park Nicollet's three geriatric nurse practitioners make joint rounds with physicians in several of these homes. The Medical Center has initiated a "preferred nursing home" program in order to improve quality and efficiency in a select smaller number of nursing homes. A key element in the nursing home model is that Park Nicollet geriatrician directs the development of preferred relationships and supervises the geriatric nurse practitioners.

Joint Venture with Local Hospital. The Park Nicollet Medical Center and the Methodist Hospital formed a joint venture to provide health maintenance at a local senior high-rise. Two registered nurses, one from Park Nicollet and one from the Hospital, visit the high-rise every other week for a two-hour period. Blood pressures are taken and health education information is shared with the residents. This program is generating referrals back to the Clinic and to the Hospital. The joint venture between the Hospital and the Clinic is evaluated annually.

Geriatric Assessment. A geriatric assessment team, comprised of two registered nurses and one social worker, provides home visits to the frail elderly. They review how well the patient is functioning and assess the environment (i.e., medicines in the medicine cabinet, food in cupboards and refrigerator, cleanliness). They also set up new medicine regimes for patients. The team reports their findings back to the medical director.

At this time, Medicare does not reimburse for this assessment. This service is paid for out of pocket by the patient.

The Duluth Clinic, Limited

The Duluth Clinic, Limited, is a large, multispecialty group practice comprised of 150 physicians. The Clinic was founded in 1915 and is structured as a not-for-profit corporation. Over 750 employees work for this group. It has initiated a number of programs to educate seniors and professionals in the community.

Health Education Presentations. The Duluth Clinic, Limited, Gerontology Department sponsors or cosponsors with other health care institutions a variety of health education seminars. Some topics presented include volunteering, caregiving, communication and aging as a family issue and Alzheimer's disease. and The Duluth Clinic Gerontology Program.

The Gift of Memories Album. The "Gift of Memories Album" was developed by The Duluth Clinic, Limited, as a resource for patients to record their life history. The album organizes different life events into separate sections. This album has been distributed to over 1,000 people in the Duluth area. Seminars on reminiscence and life review were also conducted at community request. At the present time, The Duluth Clinic, Limited, does not charge patients in their geriatric assessment and case management program for the album; however, a contribution is requested from the general public. A similar type of album could be developed by any clinic's staff and distributed to patients and families for a fee. In addition, the album can provide positive public relations for the clinic. Topics in the album include: First Memories, My Favorite Things, Childhood, Adulthood, I Remember When, My Recollection of Historical Events, Words of Wisdom, Stories and others.

Healthy Lifestyle Approaches Workbook. The "Healthy Lifestyles Approaches Workbook" is a beginning step for self-assessment of one's health. This booklet can be distributed to existing patients as well as potential patients to market the clinic. Sections include: Nutrition, Stress, Exercise, Smoking, Sleep Patterns. This booklet is similar to the "Tips for Healthy Living" booklet mentioned in Chapter III.

Aging Awareness Questionnaire. The Aging Awareness Questionnaire is used to sensitize staff to the needs of the elderly. The questionnaire, adapted from Dr. Erdman B. Palmore's Facts on Aging Quiz, is given as part of new employee orientation, as well as to long-term employees, to break down stereotypes and myths that are present in our society. Once attitudes regarding the elderly have changed, people's behavior will also change. The CRAHCA video, "In Our Age: The Older Patient," is also a useful educational tool.

Geriatric Assessment. The geriatric assessment, developed by CRAHCA, is performed by volunteer students as part of their Master's practicum. The assessment is a multidisciplinary tool used to determine activities of daily living, functional ability, social and economic resources and home environment. Volunteers from local universities, including bachelor and master candidates in social work, gerontology, psychology, nursing and health education, are trained to perform the assessment. Assessment results are reported to the primary care physician along with recommendations to maximize health and well-being.

Senior Expo Fair. The Duluth Clinic, Limited, participated in the local "Senior Expo Fair," a community-wide event which included health providers, social service agencies and for-profit corporations interested in marketing to the elderly. A booth was purchased to promote their services. The Duluth Clinic also sponsored an "Intergenerational Workshop" at the fair in conjunction with the Gerontology Consortium in the community. The consortium is comprised of Miller Dwan Medical Center, St. Mary's Medical Center, the College of St. Scholastica and The Duluth Clinic, Limited. The educational workshop promoted all the members of the consortium, generating goodwill and name recognition within the community.

Practicum Site. Students from the University of Minnesota, Duluth and the College of St. Scholastica were placed in geriatric practicums at The Duluth Clinic, Limited. The students' educational backgrounds included geropsychology, education, social work and health management/administration.

The Honolulu Medical Group

The Honolulu Medical Group is a multispecialty group with more than 50 physicians on staff which has been a leader in the field of geriatrics in Hawaii for a number of years. Founded in 1903, the practice is a free-standing professional corporation. Each of the programs implemented by this practice may also be replicated in other group practices.

Wellness Program. The Honolulu Medical Group has developed a number of wellness and health management programs, which are advertised in local community papers and a senior publication called "The Healthy Aging Project." These include:
— A *fitness exercise class* for anyone age 65 and older is offered by the Group. These classes are taught five days a week by an exercise specialist. Physicians refer individuals to this program.
— A *weekly senior lecture series* is offered on topics of health and life enrichment. The series is open to the public.

— *Preventive medicine programs* have been developed to educate patients regarding the management of chronic conditions such as diabetes, hypertension, arthritis and heart disease. New cholesterol and foot care clinics were opened in April of 1988.

BestCare Supplemental Insurance Program. The "BestCare Supplemental Insurance Program" evolved out of a joint venture between the Honolulu Medical Group, a local insurance company and a local hospital. The focus of the joint venture was to make available to the public a comprehensive senior health service at a reasonable price.

The "BestCare Supplemental Insurance Program" offers seniors a Medicare supplemental insurance policy which can only be used at the Honolulu Medical Group. The plan has enrolled 115 people and appeals to the well elderly. It is competitively priced for the Honolulu market. The Group does not consider the practices' supplemental insurance plan as a risk but uses this program to attract new patients.

Geriatric Assessments. The Honolulu Medical Group also performs geriatric assessments in the home of the frail elderly to impact their medical outcome. Physicians refer patients who are over 75 to the assessment team. The team consists of a nurse, a social worker and two volunteers with social work experience. The volunteers are both over 60. The practice has found that the interaction in the home between the patient and the volunteer is very positive. The patient tends to share more information with the volunteer because the volunteer is so close to his or her age. The volunteers report back to the team, who then follow-up. Volunteers call patients every 60 days instead of weekly as is done at Park Nicollet Medical Center. The volunteers report their findings to the case manager and document the need for further follow-up. The volunteers were recruited through an advertisement in the *Honolulu Medical Group Practice Newsletter.*

Honolulu Gerontology Program. The "Honolulu Gerontology Program" was founded by the Honolulu Medical Group Research and Education Foundation and provides the following services: 1) case management services for frail elderly patients; 2) health maintenance program which offers rehabilitative exercises, education and socialization to frail, elderly patients; 3) family caregiver support program which offers monthly caregiver support meetings and an annual eight-week caregiver educational series; and, 4) senior advisor/volunteer program which trains retired professionals to work with frail homebound elderly. The "Honolulu Gerontology Program" is offered throughout Oahu and generates name recognition and goodwill for the Honolulu Medical Group.

Comprehensive Outpatient Rehabilitation Facility (CORF) Program. The Honolulu Medical Group developed a CORF as a part of the rehabilitation component of the Senior Health Service. A CORF is primarily a Medicare-approved rehabilitation center servicing individuals 65 and older. Over 100 individuals received outpatient rehabilitation in 1988.

Educational Preceptorship and Practicum Placement Site. Students from the University of Hawaii's Graduate School of Social Work and School of Nursing have been placed at the Honolulu Medical Group for a geriatric practicum. Students assist in special projects and increase the manpower of the program to provide more direct service to patients.

Geriatric Standards and Protocols. The Honolulu Medical Group conducted a thorough review of the literature pertaining to care of persons 65 and older. Based on their findings, a manual defining the Group's standards of care was developed. Protocols were also written to correspond to the standards of care.

Carle Clinic Association

The Carle Clinic, founded in 1931, is a large multispecialty group practice in Urbana, Illinois, with over 200 physicians. Two-thirds of the physicians specialize in primary care. Thirty-eight medical and surgical specialties and subspecialties are also represented including geriatrics, cardiology, audiology, orthopaedics, oncology, otolaryngology, ophthalmology and rheumatology. Branch clinics are located in other central Illinois communities. The Carle Clinic Association is linked to Carle Foundation Hospital, The Carle Arbours continuing Long-Term Care Center and the Carle Pavilion, a specialty hospital offering programs for emotional problems, eating disorders and drug/alcohol dependence. To meet the special health care needs of older Americans, the Carle Clinic Association offers many specialized geriatric programs and services.

Geriatric Evaluation Clinic. The Geriatric Evaluation Clinic provides comprehensive evaluation services for people 65 and older. Patients are evaluated by a team which includes a geriatrician, geriatric nurse practitioner, social worker, rehabilitation specialist and other specialists depending on the needs of the patient. An individualized diagnosis and care plan is developed and returned to the patient's primary physician for review and follow-up.

Geriatric Consulting Service. The Carle Clinic Association developed the "Geriatric Consulting Service" to optimize care for the Carle's nursing home residents. A team of geriatric nurse practitioners, internists and family practitioners provide ongoing medical care for the nursing home residents.

Home Consultation Service. Nurse practitioners visit frail, elderly patients in their homes to maintain independent living, provide early detection and prevention of serious illnesses and make health care referrals as needed.

Wellness Program. Health education classes are offered in senior centers, to community groups and to banks with senior clubs. The wellness programs encourage and motivate older adults to begin and/or maintain an active healthy lifestyle. Health promotion classes, fitness programs, cholesterol screenings, health risk appraisals and consultation and referral services are offered. A caregiver seminar is a new program which the Carle Clinic will be offering to businesses during the noon hour. Many caregivers work, so Carle Clinic will teach the class at the workplace.

Senior Companion Action Grant. The Carle Clinic received an Action Grant from the federal government to train seniors on fixed incomes to be senior companions. Each senior receives 40 hours of training prior to being placed with a frail, elderly person. The senior receives $2.20/hour plus 2 weeks paid vacation. A full-time nurse was hired to administer the grant. An advisory committee made up of members of community service agencies, elderly patients and the Carle Clinic staff oversee the Action Grant program.

Alzheimer's Grant. The Carle Clinic was chosen as one of seven sites for a federally funded Medicare Alzheimer's Disease Demonstration to study how case management services can assist Alzheimer's patients. The grant services 10 neighboring counties. Alzheimer's disease screenings and case management and community-based services are provided to a study group comprised of 200 seniors. A control group receives only the screening. This grant has added to Carle Clinic's name recognition in the elderly community and among the social service agencies which serve this population.

Focus Groups. Carle Clinic Association conducted two focus groups with older residents to determine their attitudes toward health care service delivery and patient decision-making characteristics. The residents were chosen at random from a phone list and included rural and urban participants. Questions were developed by the Carle Clinic Association regarding loyalty to health care providers, source of health information and cost to name a few. The results were tabulated and shared with the staff who incorporated them into their marketing efforts.

Dementia Drug Trials. Carle Clinic is a site for two multicenter trials of new medication for patients with dementia of the Alzheimer's type. Patients receive medication and all procedures associated with the study free of charge. Their progress is monitored regularly by Carle Clinic physicians.

Carle Outreach Program for the Elderly (COPE). COPE is a case management program which assists senior adults in their efforts to live independently at home. A case manager administers a comprehensive in-home assessment, evaluates client health and daily living needs and develops a plan of care. On an ongoing basis, the case manager can make referrals to appropriate Carle/community resources, coordinate service delivery and address patient concerns. The case manager also maintains contact with the patient's primary physician.

APPENDIX 1
Part B Medicare Insurance Carriers

Alabama
Medicare Blue Cross Blue Shield of
 Alabama
P. O. Box C 140
Birmingham, Alabama 35205

Alaska
Medicare
Aetna Life & Casualty
Crown Plaza
1500 S.W. First Avenue
Portland, Oregon 97201
Wallingford, CT 06493

Arizona
Medicare
Aetna Life & Casualty
Medicare Claim Administration
3010 West Fairmount Avenue
Phoenix, Arizona 85017

Arkansas
Medicare
Arkansas Blue Cross and Blue Shield
P. O. Box 1418
Little Rock, Arkansas 72203

California
Counties of: Los Angeles, Orange, San
 Diego, Ventura, Imperial, San Luis
 Obispo, Santa Barbara:
Medicare
Transamerica Occidental Life
 Insurance Company
Box 54905
Terminal Annex
Los Angeles, California 90054
Executive Park Station

Rest of California:
Medicare Claims Department
Blue Shield of California
Chico, California 95976

Colorado
Medicare
Blue Shield of Colorado
700 Broadway
Denver, Colorado 80273

Connecticut
Medicare
Connecticut General Life Insurance
 Company
100 Barnes Road, North
P. O. Box 5005

Delaware
Medicare
Pennsylvania Blue Shield
P. O. Box 65
Camp Hill, PA 17011

District of Columbia
Medicare
Pennsylvania Blue Shield
P. O. Box 100
Camp Hill, Pennsylvania 17011

Florida
Medicare
Blue Shield of Florida
P. O. Box 2525
Jacksonville, Florida 32231

Appendix 1

Georgia
The Prudential Insurance Co. of America
Medicare Part B
P. O. Box 546
Buford, Georgia 30518

Hawaii
Medicare
Aetna Life and Casualty
P. O. Box 3947
Honolulu, Hawaii 96812

Idaho
Medicare
The Equitable Life Assurance Society
P. O. Box 8048
Boise, Idaho 83707

Illinois
E.D.S. Federal Corp.
Medicare Claims
P. O. Box 4422
Marion, Illinois 62959

Indiana
Medicare Part B
120 West Market Street
Indianapolis, Indiana 46204

Iowa
Medicare
Blue Shield of Iowa
636 Grand
Des Moines, Iowa 50307

Kansas
Counties of: Johnson, Wyandotte
Medicare
Blue Shield of Kansas City
P. O. Box 169
Kansas City, Missouri 64141

Rest of Kansas:
Medicare
Blue Shield of Kansas
P. O. Box 239
Topeka, Kansas 66601

Kentucky
Medicare Part B
Blue Cross and Blue Shield of Kentucky
1218 Harrodsburg Road
Lexington, Kentucky 40504

Louisiana
Medicare
Pan American Life Insurance Co.
P. O. Box 60450
New Orleans, Louisiana 70160

Maine
Medicare
Blue Shield of Massachusetts- Maine
P. O. Box 1010
Biddeford, Maine 04005

Maryland
Counties of: Montgomery, Prince Georges
Medicare
Pennsylvania Blue Shield
P. O. Box 100
Camp Hill, Pennsylvania 17011

Rest of Maryland:
Maryland Blue Shield, Inc.
700 East Joppa Road
Towson, Maryland 21204

Massachusetts
Medicare
Blue Shield of Massachusetts, Inc.
55 Accord Park Drive
Rockland, Massachusetts 02371

Michigan
Medicare
Blue Shield of Michigan
P. O. Box 2201
Detroit, Michigan 48231

Minnesota
Counties of: Anoka, Dakota Filmore,
   Goodhue, Hennepin Houston, Olmstead,
   Ramsey, Wabasha, Washington, Winona:
Medicare
The Travelers Insurance Co.
8120 Penn Avenue, South
Bloomington, Minnesota 55431

Rest of Minnesota:
Medicare
Blue Shield of Minnesota
P. O. Box 43357
St. Paul, Minnesota 55164

Mississippi
Medicare
The Travelers Insurance Co.
P. O. Box 22545
Jackson, Mississippi 39205

Missouri
Counties of: Andrew, Atchison, Bates,
   Benton, Buchanan, Caldwell Carroll,
   Cass, Clay, Clinton, Daviess, DeKalb,
   Gentry, Grundy, Harrison, Henry, Holt,
   Jackson, Johnson, Lafayette, Livingston,
   Mercer, Nodaway, Pettis, Platte, Ray, St.
   Clair, Saline, Vernon, Worth:
Medicare
Blue Shield of Kansas City
P. O. Box 169
Kansas City, Missouri 64141

Rest of Missouri:
Medicare
Gen'l American Life Ins. Co.
P. O. Box 505
St. Louis, Missouri 63166

Montana
Medicare
Montana Physicians' Service
P. O. Box 4310
Helena, Montana 59601

Nebraska
Medicare
Mutual of Omaha Insurance Co.
P. O. Box 456, Downtown Station
Omaha, Nebraska 68101

Nevada
Medicare
Aetna Life & Casualty
P. O. Box 11260
Phoenix, Arizona 85017

New Hampshire
Medicare
New Hampshire-Vermont
Physician Service
Two Pillsbury Street
Concord, New Hampshire 03306

New Jersey
Medicare
The Prudential Insurance Co. of America
P. O. Box 3000
Linwood, New Jersey 08221

New Mexico
Medicare
The Equitable Life Assurance Soc.
P. O. Box 3070, Station D
Albuquerque, New Mexico 87110

New York
Counties of: Bronx, Columbia Delaware, Dutchess, Greene, Kings, Nassau, New York, Orange, Putman, Richmond, Rockland, Suffolk, Sullivan, Ulster, Westchester:
Medicare
BC/BS of Greater New York
P. O. Box 458
Murray Hill Station
New York, New York 10016

County of Queens:
Medicare
Group Health, Inc.
P. O. Box A966
Times Square Station
New York, New York 10036

Rest of New York:
Medicare
Blue Shield of Western New York
P. O. Box 600
Binghamton, New York 13902

North Carolina
The Prudential Insurance Company of America
Medicare B Division
P. O. Box 2126
High Point, North Carolina 27261

North Dakota
Medicare
Blue Shield of North Dakota
4510 13th Avenue, S.W.
Fargo, North Dakota 58121

Ohio
Medicare
Nationwide Mutual Insurance Co.
P. O. Box 57
Columbus, Ohio 43216

Oklahoma
Medicare
Aetna Life & Casualty
Jamestown Office Park
3031 N.W. 64th Street
Oklahoma City, Oklahoma 73116

Oregon
Medicare
Aetna Life and Casualty
Crown Plaza
1500 S.W. First Avenue
Portland, Oregon 97201

Pennsylvania
Medicare
Pennsylvania Blue Shield
Box 65 Blue Shield Building
Camp Hill, Pennsylvania 17011

Rhode Island
Medicare
Blue Shield of Rhode Island
444 Westminster Mall
Providence, Rhode Island 02901

South Carolina
Medicare
Blue Shield of South Carolina
Drawer F, Forest Acres Branch
Columbia, South Carolina 29260

South Dakota
Medicare
Blue Shield of North Dakota
4510 13th Avenue, S.W.
Fargo, North Dakota 58121

Tennessee
Medicare
The Equitable Life Assurance Soc.
P. O. Box 1465
Nashville, Tennessee 37202

Texas
Medicare
Group Medical and Surgical Service
P. O. Box 222147
Dallas, Texas 75222

Utah
Medicare
BC/BS of Utah
P. O. Box 30270
2455 Parley's Way
Salt Lake City, Utah 84125

Vermont
Medicare
New Hampshire-Vermont
Physician Service
Two Pillsbury Street
Concord, New Hampshire 03306

Virginia
Counties of: Arlington, Fairfax
Cities of: Alexandria, Falls Church, Fairfax:
Medicare
Pennsylvania Blue Shield
P. O. Box 100
Camp Hill, Pennsylvania 17011

Washington
Medicare
Washington Physicians' Service
Mail to your local Medical Service Bureau.
 (If you do not know which bureau handles your claim, mail to:
Medicare Washington
Physicians' Service
4th and Battery Bldg.
6th Floor
2401 4th Avenue
Seattle, Washington 98121

West Virginia
Medicare
Nationwide Mutual Insurance Co.
P. O. Box 57
Columbus, Ohio 43216

Wisconsin
Medicare
Wisc. Physicians' Service
Box 1787
Madison, Wisconsin 53701

Wyoming
Medicare
The Equitable Life Assurance Soc.
P. O. Box 628
Cheyenne, Wyoming 82001

APPENDIX 2
Referral Agencies

STATE AGENCIES ON AGING — Refer to the State Agency on Aging for your local Area Agency on Aging (AAA) chapter.

ALABAMA
STATE AGENCY ON AGING
COMMISSION ON AGING DIVISION
136 Catoma Street
Montgomery, Alabama 36130
(205) 261-5743

ALASKA
OLDER ALASKANS COMMISSION
Department of Administration
Pouch C-Mail Station 0209
Juneau, Alaska 99811
(907) 465-3250

ARIZONA
STATE AGENCY ON AGING AGING AND
 ADULT ADMINISTRATION/Department of
 Economic Security
1400 West Washington Street
Phoenix, Arizona 85007
Office: (602) 255-4446
I & R #: (800)-352-3792 (AZ only)

ARKANSAS
STATE AGENCY ON AGING
OFFICE OF AGING AND ADULT
 SERVICES
7th and Main Streets
Donaghey Building - Suite 1417
Little Rock, Arkansas 72201
(501) 682-2441

CALIFORNIA
STATE AGENCY ON AGING
DEPARTMENT ON AGING
1600 K Street
Sacramento, California 95814
Office: (916)-322-3887

COLORADO
STATE AGENCY ON AGING
AGING AND ADULT SERVICES DIVISION
1575 Sherman
Denver, Colorado 80218-0899
(303) 866-5905

CONNECTICUT
STATE AGENCY ON AGING
DEPARTMENT ON AGING
175 Main Street
Hartford, Connecticut 06106
Office: (203) 566-3238
I&R #: (800) 443-9946 (CT only)

DELAWARE
DIVISION ON AGING
Department of Health and Human Services
1901 North Dupont Highway
New Castle, Delaware 19720
Office: (302) 421-6791
I&R #: (800) 223-9074 (DE only)

DISTRICT OF COLUMBIA
OFFICE ON AGING
1424 K Street, N.W.
2nd Floor
Washington, DC 20005
Office: (202) 724-5626
I&R #: (202) 724-5626

FLORIDA
STATE AGENCY ON AGING
Department of Health and Rehabilitative
   Services
1317 Winewood Blvd.
Tallahassee, Florida 32301
Office: (904) 488-8922
I&R #: (800) 342-0825 (FL only)

GEORGIA
STATE AGENCY ON AGING
OFFICE OF AGING
878 Peachtree Street, N.E.
Room #632
Atlanta, GA 30309
(404) 894-5333

HAWAII
STATE AGENCY ON AGING
EXECUTIVE OFFICE OF AGING
335 Merchant Street
Room #241
Honolulu, Hawaii 96813
(808) 548-2593

IDAHO
STATE AGENCY ON AGING
IDAHO OFFICE ON AGING
Room 114 Statehouse
Boise, Idaho 83720
Office: (208) 334-3833
I&R #: (208) 378-0111

ILLINOIS
STATE AGENCY ON AGING
DEPARTMENT OF AGING
421 East Capitol Avenue
Springfield, Illinois 62701
Office: (217) 785-2870
I&R #: (800) 252-8966 (IL only)

INDIANA
STATE AGENCY ON AGING
COMMISSION ON AGING & AGED
251 N. Illinois St./POB 7083
Indianapolis, Indiana 46207
Office: (317) 232-7006
I&R #: (800) 622-4972 (IN only)

IOWA
STATE AGENCY ON AGING
IOWA DEPARTMENT OF ELDER AFFAIRS
914 Grand Avenue #236
Des Moines, Iowa 50319
Office: (515) 281-5187
I&R #: (800) 532-3213 (IA only)

KANSAS
STATE AGENCY ON AGING
DEPARTMENT ON AGING
610 West Tenth
Topeka, Kansas 66612
Office: (913) 296-4986
I&R #: (800)-432-3535 (KS only)

KENTUCKY
STATE AGENCY ON AGING
DIVISION FOR AGING SERVICES
275 E. Main Street
Frankfort, KY 40601
(502) 564-6930

LOUISIANA
STATE AGENCY ON AGING
OFFICE OF ELDERLY AFFAIRS
4528 Remington Avenue
P. O. Box 80374
Baton Rouge, LA 70898
(504) 925-1700

MAINE
STATE AGENCY ON AGING
BUREAU OF MAINE'S ELDERLY
State House #11
Augusta, Maine 04333
(207) 289-2561

MARYLAND
STATE AGENCY ON AGING
OFFICE ON AGING
301 W. Preston St., #1004
Baltimore, Maryland 21201
Office: (301) 225-1100
I&R #: (800)-338-0153 (MD only)

MASSACHUSETTS
STATE AGENCY ON AGING
EXECUTIVE OFFICE OF ELDER AFFAIRS
38 Chauncy Street
Boston, Massachusetts 02111
Office: (617) 727-7750
I&R #: (800) 882-2003

MICHIGAN
STATE AGENCY ON AGING
OFFICE OF SERVICES TO THE AGING
300 E. Michigan Avenue
P. O. Box 30026
Lansing, Michigan 48909
(517) 373-8230

MINNESOTA
STATE AGENCY ON AGING
MINNESOTA BOARD ON AGING
444 Lafayette Road, 4th Floor
St. Paul, Minnesota 55155
Office: (612) 296-2544
I&R #: (800) 652-9747

MISSISSIPPI
STATE AGENCY ON AGING
MISSISSIPPI COUNCIL ON AGING
301 West Pearl Street
Jackson, Mississippi 39203
Office: (601) 949-2070
I&R #: (800) 222-7622 (MS only)

MISSOURI
STATE AGENCY ON AGING
DEPARTMENT OF SOCIAL SERVICES - DIV. ON AGING
2701 W. Main Street
Jefferson City, Missouri 65102
Office: (314) 751-3082
I&R #: (800) 235-5503 (MO only)

MONTANA
STATE AGENCY ON AGING
DEPARTMENT OF FAMILY SERVICES
PO Box 8005/48 North Last Chance Gulch
Helena, Montana 59604
Office: (406) 444-5900
I&R #: (800) 332-2272 (MT only)

NEBRASKA
STATE AGENCY ON AGING
DEPARTMENT ON AGING
301 Centennial Mall So.
PO Box 95044
Lincoln, Nebraska 68509
(402) 471-2306

NEVADA
DIVISION FOR AGING SERVICES
505 East King Street, #101
Carson City, Nevada 89710
Office: (702) 885-4210
I&R #: (702) 885-4210

NEW HAMPSHIRE
DIVISION OF ELDERLY AND ADULT
    SERVICES
6 Hazen Drive
Concord, New Hampshire 03301
Office: (603) 271-4394
I&R #: (800) 852-3345 (NH only)

NEW JERSEY
STATE AGENCY ON AGING
DIVISION ON AGING
DEPARTMENT OF COMMUNITY AFFAIRS
    CN 807
South Broad and Front Streets
Trenton, New Jersey 08625
Office: (609) 292-4833
I&R #: (800) 792-8820 (NJ only)

NEW MEXICO
STATE AGENCY ON AGING
224 East Palace Avenue, 4th Floor
Santa Fe, New Mexico 87501
Office: (505) 827-7640
I&R #: (800) 432-2080 (NM only)

NEW YORK
STATE AGENCY ON AGING
OFFICE FOR THE AGING
Empire State Plaza, Building #2
Albany, New York 12223
Office: (518) 474-4425
I&R #: (800) 342-9871 (NY only)

NORTH CAROLINA
STATE AGENCY ON AGING
DIVISION ON AGING
1985 Umpstead Drive, Kirby Bldg.
Raleigh, North Carolina 27603
Office: (919) 733-3983
I&R #: (800) 662-7030 (NC only)

NORTH DAKOTA
AGING SERVICES/DEPT. OF HUMAN
    SERVICES
State Capitol Building
Bismarck, North Dakota 58505
Office: (701) 224-2577
I&R #: (800) 472-2622 (ND only)

OHIO
STATE AGENCY ON AGING
DEPARTMENT ON AGING
50 West Broad Street, 9th Floor
Columbus, Ohio 43266
(614) 466-5500

OKLAHOMA
STATE AGENCY ON AGING
SPECIAL UNIT ON AGING
P. O. Box 25352
Oklahoma City, Oklahoma 73125
(405) 521-2281

OREGON
STATE AGENCY ON AGING
SENIOR SERVICES DIVISION
313 Public Service Building
Salem, Oregon 97310
(503) 378-4728

Appendix 2

PENNSYLVANIA
STATE AGENCY ON AGING
DEPARTMENT OF AGING
231 State Street, #307
Harrisburg, PA 17101-1195
(717) 783-1550

RHODE ISLAND
DEPARTMENT OF ELDERLY AFFAIRS
79 Washington Street
Providence, Rhode Island 02903
Office: (401) 277-2858
I&R #: (800) 752-8088 (RI only)

SOUTH CAROLINA
STATE AGECNY ON AGING
COMMISSION ON AGING
400 Arbor Lake Drive #B-500
Columbia, South Carolina 29223
(803) 735-0210

SOUTH DAKOTA
OFFICE OF ADULT SERVICES & AGING
700 Governors Drive, Kneip Bldg.
Pierre, South Dakota 57501
Office: (605) 773-3656
I&R #: (605) 975-2222 (SD only)

TENNESSEE
STATE AGENCY ON AGING
COMMISSION ON AGING
706 Church Street, #201
Nashville, Tennessee 37219
(615) 741-2056

TEXAS
STATE AGENCY ON AGING
TEXAS DEPARTMENT OF AGING
1949 IH 35, South
Austin, Texas 78741-3702
Office: (512) 444-2727
I&R #: (800) 252-9240 (TX only)

UTAH
STATE AGENCY ON AGING
DIVISION OF AGING AND ADULT
  SERVICES
120 North 200 West
P. O. Box 45500
Salt Lake City, Utah 84145-0500
(801) 538-3910

VERMONT
STATE AGENCY ON AGING
OFFICE ON AGING
103 South Main Street
Waterbury, Vermont 05676
Office: (802) 241-2400
I&R #: (800) 642-5119

VIRGINIA
STATE AGENCY ON AGING
DEPARTMENT OF AGING
700 E. Franklin Street
10th Floor
Richmond, Virginia 23219
Office: (804) 225-2271
I&R #: (800) 55-AGING (VA only)

WASHINGTON
STATE AGENCY ON AGING
AGING AND ADULT SERVICES
  ADMINISTRATION
OB-44A
Olympia, Washington 98504
Office: (206) 586-3768
I&R #: (800) 422-3263 (WA only)

WEST VIRGINIA
STATE AGENCY ON AGING
COMMISSION ON AGING
Holly Grove - State Capitol
Charleston, West Virginia 25305
Office: (304) 348-3317
I&R #: (800) 642-3671

WISCONSIN
STATE AGENCY ON AGING
BUREAU ON AGING
217 South Hamilton St. #300
Madison, Wisconsin 53703
(608) 266-2536

WYOMING
STATE OFFICE ON AGING
720 W. 18 St. Hathaway Bldg. #139
Cheyenne, Wyoming 82002
Office: (307) 777-7986
I&R #: (307) 777-7986

Other Resource Agencies

Adult Daycare

National Institute on Adult Daycare
600 Maryland Avenue S.W.
West Wing 100
Washington, DC 20024
(202) 479-1200

Alcohol and Drug Abuse

National Clearinghouse for Alcohol
 and Drug Information
P. O. Box 2345
Rockeville, Maryland 20852
(301) 468-2600

Alzheimer's Disease

Alzheimer's Disease and Related
 Disorders Association (Nat'l)
70 E. Lake Street, Suite 600
Chicago, Illinois 60601
(312) 853-3060

Blindness

National Society to Prevent Blindness
500 E. Remington Road
Schaumburg, Illinois 60173
(312) 843-2020

Blindness (continued)

American Council for the Blind
1010 Vermont Rd. W., Suite 1100
Washington, DC 20005
(202) 393-3666
(800) 424-8666

National Library Service for the Blind and
 Physically Handicapped
1291 Taylor Street
Washington, DC 20542
(800) 424-8567
(202) 287-5100

Hearing Disorders

The Nat'l Information Center on Deafness
Gallaudet College
800 Florida Avenue N.E.
Washington, DC 20002
(202) 651-5109

The National Association for Hearing and
 Speech Action
10801 Rockville Pike
Rockville, Maryland 20852
(301) 897-8682

Appendix 2

Home Health/Home Care

American Federation of Home Health Care Agencies
1320 Fenwick Lane
Silver Spring, Maryland 20910
(301) 588-1454

National Association of Home Care
519 C Street N.E.
Washington, DC 20002
(202) 547-7424

Hospice

Hospice Education Institute
P. O. Box 713
Essex, Connecticut 06426
(800) 331-1620

National Hospice Organization
901 N. Moore Street, Suite 901
Arlington, Virginia 22209
(703) 243-5900

Housing

American Association of Homes for the Aging
1129 20th Street, N.W.
Suite 400
Washington, DC 20036
(202) 296-5960

Legal Issues

National Senior Citizens Law Center
2028 M Street N.W.
Suite 400
Washington, DC 20036
(202) 887-5280

Long Term Care

National Center for State Long Term Care Ombudsman Resources
2033 K Street NW
Suite 304
Washington, DC 20006
(202) 785-0707

Mental Health

National Institute of Mental Health
U. S. Department of Human Services
5600 Fischers Lane
Room 15C-05
Rockville, Maryland 20857
(301) 443-4513

Victims Assistance

National Organization for Victim Assistance
717 David Street N.W.
Washington, D.C 20004
(202) 393-6682

National Victims Center
307 W. 7th Street
Suite 1001
Fort Worth, Texas 76102
(817) 877-3355

Widowed Persons

Widowed Persons Service
1909 K Street N.W.
Washington, DC 20049
(202)-728-4370

General Agencies

American Association of Retired Persons (AARP)
1909 K Street N.W.
Washington, DC 20049
(800) 523-5800

American Red Cross National Headquarters
18th and D Street N.W.
Washington, DC 20006
(202) 737-8300

Food and Drug Administration
Frank Young, M.D.,Ph.D., Commissioner
Rockville, MD 20857
(301) 443-2410

National Council on Aging
600 Maryland Avenue S.W.
WW100
Washington, DC 20024
(800) 424-9046
(202) 479-1200

National Institute on Aging
9000 Rockville Pike, Building 31
Bethesda, Maryland 20014
(301) 496-1752

General Agencies (continued)

Social Security Administration
Dorcas R. Hardy, Commissioner
Baltimore, Maryland 21235
(301) 965-8882

United Way of America
701 N. Fairfax Street
Alexandria, Virginia 22314
(703) 836-7100

U.S. Department of Health and Human Services
Office of Disease Prevention and Health Promotion
Washington, DC 20201
(202) 245-7611

Volunteers of America
3813 N. Causeway Boulevard
Metairie, Louisiana 70002
(504) 837-2652

BIBLIOGRAPHY

Barrow, Georgia M. and Patricia A. Smith. *Aging, Agism and Society.* St. Paul, Minnesota: West Publishing Company, 1979.

Berenson, Robert A. "A Physician's Perspective on Case Management." *Business and Health* July/August 1985, 22-25.

Bergstrom, Anna M. "Case Management of Frail Elders in Medical Group Practices." *Generations* Fall 1987, 54-56.

Crump, William J., M.D. "Who Lives? Who Dies? What the Courts are Saying about Living Wills." *Senior Patient* March/April 1989, 76-83.

Crump, William J., M.D. "Who Lives? Who Dies? Who Decides? Helping Your Patient Prepare a Living Will." *Senior Patient* March/April 1989, 85-92.

Dychwald, Dr. Ken and Mark Zitter. *The Role of a Hospital in an Aging Society: A Blueprint for Action.* San Francisco: Age Wave, 1986.

Grey, Hilda, DPA. "Geriatrics - An Eye for the Future." *Journal of the Medical Group Management Association* May/June 1986, 14-16, 33.

Haug, Marie R., Ph.D., Editor. *Elderly Patients and Their Doctors.* New York, New York: Springer Publishing Co., 1981.

Hiatt, Lorraine G. "Effective Design for Informal Conversation." *American Health Care Association Journal* 1983, 9 (2), 43-46.

Hiatt, Lorraine G. "Conveying the Substance of Images, Interior Design in Long-Term Care." *Contemporary Administrator* April 1984, 17.

Hiatt, Lorraine G. "Environmental Design and the Frail Older Person at Home."

Hiatt, Lorraine G. "The Color and Use of Color in Environments for Older People." *Nursing Homes* 1981, 30 (3), 18-22.

Hiatt, Lorraine G. "The Happy Wanderer." *Nursing Homes* 1980, 29 (2), 27-31.

Hiatt, Lorraine G. "Designing Therapeutic Dining." *Nursing Homes* March/April 1981, 30 (2), 33-39.

Hiatt, Lorraine G. "Living Environments, Geriatric Wheelchairs and Older Persons' Rehabilitation." *Journal of Gerontological Nursing* Nov/Dec 1975, 1 (5), 17-20.

Hiatt, Lorraine G. "Disorientation is More than a State of Mind." *Nursing Homes* 1980, 29 (4), 30-36.

Hiatt, Lorraine G., Ph.D. "Environmental Design Report to St. Mary's Hospital."

Hiatt, Lorraine G., Ph.D. "The Importance of the Physical Environment." *Nursing Homes* September/October 1982, 31 (4), 2-10.

Hiatt, Lorraine G. "Understanding the Physical Environment." *Pride Institute Journal* 1985, 4 (2), 12-22.

Huttman, Elizabeth D. *Social Services for the Elderly* New York, New York: The Free Press, 1985.

Jahnigen, Dennis, "The Changing Doctor-Patient Relationship." *Generations* Fall 1987, 54-56.

Kimble, Cathy Stauffer and Mary E. Longe *Health Promotion Programs for Older Adults.* American Hospital Publishing, Inc., 1987.

Kline, Donald, Ph.D., Dean of School Psychology, University of Calgary, Calgary, Alberta, Canada, Interview, September 16, 1988, *Health Care Financing Review.* (Fall 1988) 10(1), "To Sign or Not to Sign: Physician Participation in Medicare, 1984" by Janet B. Mitchell, Margo L. Rosenbach and Jerry Cromwell, 17-25.

Landaw, I. "Beyond Medicare." *Consumer Reports* June 1989.

Nodar, Richard H. "Hearing Loss and Hearing Aids." *Generations* Fall 1987, 39-40.

Palmore, Erdman B., Ph.D. *The Facts on Aging Quiz* New York, New York: Springer.

Pease, Joan A. "Carpeting." *Generations* Fall 1986, 11 (1): 41-44.

Pegels, C. Carl, Ph.D. *Health Care and the Older Citizen* Rockville, Maryland: Aspen Publishers, Inc., 1988.

Poniatowski, Lisa, "Reducing Acute-Care Needs." *HMQ* Second Quarter 1988, 6-7.

Read, William A. "Assuring the Quality of Hospital and Physician Care." *Generations* Winter 1989, 21-25.

Schnall, Vicki L. "Growing Older: Sensory Changes." School of Home Economics, Oregon State University, April 1983.

Smith, Kenneth Brommel, "Changing Needs: Geriatric Education for Physicians." *The Aging Connection* June/July 1988, 5-12.

Solomon, David H. M.D.; Howard L. Judd, M.D.; Herbert C. Sier, M.D.; Laurence Z. M.D.; John E. Morley, M.D. "New Issues in Geriatric Care." UCLA Conference, *Annals of Internal Medicine* May 1988, 108 (3), 718-729

Sonnenschein, Mary Anne and Rocky Stone. "Can Your Hear Me?" *Generations* Fall 1986, 39-40.

Steinberg, Raymond M. and Genevieve W. Carter. *Case Management and the Elderly* Lexington, Massachusetts: Lexington Books, 1986.

Waller, Julian A. "The Older Driver." *Generations* Fall 1986, 36-37.

Index

Abuse, 41-42
Acoustics, 44
Activities of Daily Living (ADLS), 33
Adult day care, 34
Adult protection services, 42
Advertising, 53-57
Agency on Aging, 34-43, 81-86
Aging Awareness Questionnaire, 72
Alcoholics Anonymous, 43
Alzheimer's disease, 34, 75
Alzheimers Disease and Related
  Disorders Association, 86
American Association of Homes for the
  Aging, 35, 36, 87
American Association of Retired Persons,
  23, 58, 88
American Council of the Blind, 42, 86
American Federation of Home Health
  Care Agencies, 37, 43, 87
American Health Association, 58
American Red Cross, 88
American Stroke Association, 58
Appointment scheduling, 3-4
Art, 50
Assessment, 72-74
Association of Driver Educators for the
  Disabled, 64

Berenson, Robert A., 33
BestCare, 73
Billing, 8-11
Blind, 42
Business and Health, 33

Carle Outreach Program for the Elderly
  (COPE), 75
Cards, 59

Carle Clinic Association, 69, 74-75
Carpeting, 47-48
Case Management, 33, 71-75
  flow sheet, 20, 22
Center for Research in Ambulatory Health
  Care Association, 20, 25, 33, 69
Color, use of, 46-47
Communicating with the elderly, 1-4, 5
  telephone, 5
Comprehensive Outpatient Rehabilitation
  Facility (CORF), 73
Counseling, 39, 74
  insurance, 41
Crime victim, 42

Day care, See adult day care
Deaf, See hearing impaired
Demographics, 52-53
Dental care, 42
Design, See facility design
Diabetes, 42
Direct mail, 54-55
Driver's license, revocation, 64-65
Duluth Clinic Limited, The, 25, 69, 71-72
Durable power of attorney, 61

Education, See patient education
Emergency care, 42
Emergency response system, 43
Employment, 38
Encyclopedia of Social Work, 33
Equipment, 17-19, 43
Ethical issues, 61-68
Exercise program, 70-71, 72

Index

Facility design, 44-51
    acoustics, 44
    art, 50
    carpeting, 47-48
    color, use of, 46
    flooring, 47
    furniture, 48-49
    grab rails, 48
    lighting, 45
    lobby, 50
    signage, 51
Facts on Aging Quiz, 71
Fairs, See health fairs
Family support networks, 34
Flashers, 16
Flooring, 47
Focus groups, 75
Food and Drug Administration, 88
Food stamps, 41
Friendly Caller Program, 69-70
Furniture, 48-49

GeriMed of America, 24
Gift of Memories Album, 71
Gifts, 59
Glare, 44
Grab rails, 48
Grocery delivery, 37
Guardianship, 62-64

Handbook, See under patient education
HCFA 1500, 14
HCFA 1561, 12
HCFA 1561-A, 13
Health fairs, 57-58, 72
Healthy Lifestyle Approaches, 25, 31-32, 71
Hearing aids, 15-16
Hearing impaired, 6, 15-16, 43
Hearing screenings, 16
Home health agency, 34
Home health care, 43, 74

Homemakers, 34, 37, 43
Home meals, 34
Honolulu Medical Group, The, 69, 72-74
Hospice, 34
Hospice Education Institute, 34, 87
Housecleaning, 37
Housing, 36
    assisted living, 36
    independent living, 36
    nursing homes, 36, 70

Illumination, 45
Incontinence, 16
Interior design, See facility design

Joint venture, 70-71

Kellogg, W. K., Foundation, 25, 69

Legal assistance, 41
Legal issues, 61-68
Lighting, 45
Listen-box, 16
Living wills, 61-62, 66
Lobby, 50

Market research, 52-53
Marketing, 52-60, 75
    advertising, 53-57
    focus groups, 75
    market research, 52-53
Meals, 34, 36, 37, 58
Meals on Wheels, 58
Media, 53-57
Medicaid, 41
Medical equipment, See equipment
Medical Group Management Association, 69
Medical records, 19-20
Medicare, 8-11, 16, 41
    assignment, 9-10
    insurance carriers, 76-80
    part A, 10

Medicare (continued)
  part B, 10
  process, 10
  supplemental insurance, 10-11
Medications
  monitoring, 16-17
Mental health, 39-40
  centers, 39

National Association for Hearing and Speech Action, 43, 86
National Association for Home Care, 34, 37, 43, 87
National Center for State Long Term Care Ombudsman Resources, 87
National Clearing House for Alcohol and Drug Information, 43, 86
National Council on Aging, 88
National Hospice Organization, 34, 87
National Information Center on Deafness, 43, 86
National Institute on Adult Day Care, 34, 86
National Institute on Aging, 88
National Institute of Mental Health, 39, 87
National Library Service for the Blind and Physically Handicapped, 86
National Organization for Victim Assistance, 87
National Senior Citizens Law Center, 87
National Society to Prevent Blindness, 42, 86
National Victims Center, 87
Newsletters, 26
Noise, 44
Nursing homes, 36, 70
Nutrition, 43

Old Age Survivors and Disabled Income, 41
Over 50 and Fit, 70

Palmore, Erdman, 71
Pamphlets, See under patient education
Park Nicollet Medical Center, 69-71
Patient contact, 1-6
Patient education, 23-32, 71-75
  classes, 24, 58, 71, 72
  handbook, 24-25, 28-30
  handouts, 23, 27, 31-32, 71
  newsletters, 26
  pamphlets, 23, 27
Patient information booklet, 24-25, 28-30
Patient relations, 1-14
Patient satisfaction questionnaire, See questionnaire
Practicums, 72, 74
Psychiatry, 39-40
  hospital, 40
Public Service announcements, 56

Questionnaires
  patient satisfaction, 6-7

Radio, 55-56, 60
Reception area, 3-4
Referrals, 33-43
Respite care, 34-35
Retired Senior Volunteer Program (RSVP), 39
Retired Teachers Association, 58

Scheduling, See appointment scheduling
Senior centers, 38
Senior Companion Action Grant, 75
Senior companions, 35
Senior Expo Fair, 72
72-hour hold, 42
Signage, 51, 57
Social contact, 37-39, 69-70, 75
Social security, 41, 88
Social Services, 37, 41
Social workers, 39
Society for the Right to Die, 61
Speaking engagements, 58